INSIDE LYME: AN EXPERT'S GUIDE TO THE SCIENCE OF LYME DISEASE

DR. DANIEL CAMERON

ALL THINGS LYME PRESS

CONTENTS

About the Author   xi

Medical disclaimer   1
Foreword   5
Preface   7
Organization of the book   13

SECTION 1. WHERE ARE THE TICKS

1. Rapid expansion of ticks into new areas of the United States   17
2. Ticks may be in areas where they have not been seen   19
3. Evaluating the risk of tick bites at outdoor events   20
4. "Urban" ticks found in England and Chicago   23
5. Melting pot of tickborne pathogens in European hedgehogs   25
6. Deer ticks always migrating   27
7. Birds carry ticks from U.S. into Canada, and from Central America into U.S.   29
8. Novel way to track ticks in Canada with digital images   31
9. Established black-legged tick populations in Texas   34
10. Findings from a real-time assay of five tickborne pathogens   36
11. Infected ticks in the South as early as 1991   38

SECTION II. WHERE ARE THE TICKBORNE DISEASES?

12. Using dogs to map Lyme disease   43
13. Lyme disease cases jump in the southern United States   46

14. Case study: Entomologist ill after dragging for ticks in Georgia — 48
15. Lyme disease in the Southeast since 1991 — 50
16. Culture evidence of Borrelia in the southeastern U.S. after treatment — 52
17. Lyme disease underreported in Tennessee — 54
18. Lyme disease epidemic in Ohio — 55

SECTION III. CO-INFECTIONS IN TICKS.

19. Coinfections in ticks — 59
20. Coinfections of ticks are the rule — 60
21. Babesia becomes the No. 2 tickborne illness — 62
22. Babesia a growing concern for blood banks — 64
23. Half of patients with Babesia symptomatic for more than three months — 66
24. Case study: Seven-year-old boy in Manitoba has Babesia — 68
25. B. miyamotoi is the latest underdiagnosed tickborne disease — 70
26. High frequency of B. miyamotoi reported — 72
27. Pathologists at Mayo Clinic identify Borrelia mayonii from six patients — 74

SECTION IV. COMPLICATIONS OF TICKBORNE DISEASES

28. Landmark study of chronic neurologic Lyme disease — 79
29. Known complications of Lyme disease growing — 83
30. Eye problems from Lyme and other tickborne diseases on upswing — 85
31. Case study: 44-year-old has hemifacial spasm for five years — 88
32. Lyme-like disease or Baggio-Yoshinari syndrome in Brazil — 90
33. Vocal cord paralysis and Lyme disease — 93
34. Loss of libido and Lyme disease — 95
35. Case study: 59-year-old with mitral valve involvement and conduction disease — 96
36. Case study: Myocarditis in a 15-year-old adolescent — 98

37. Postmortem findings explored for five patients who died of Lyme carditis — 100
38. Case study: Diplopia and heart block in early-disseminated Lyme disease — 103
39. Case study: Physician with Lyme disease thrives after heart transplant — 105
40. Case study: 18-year-old man dies from Lyme carditis — 107
41. Case study: 79-year-old with Lyme meningitis, manifesting as Parkinson's disease — 109
42. Case study: Lyme disease with subacute parkinsonism and abnormal DaT scans — 111
43. Stroke manifestations of Lyme disease — 114
44. Case study: 43-year-old has cognitive issues following a stroke — 116
45. Case study: Kris Kristofferson's dementia was undiagnosed Lyme disease — 118
46. Case study: Two more patients with reversible Lyme disease dementia — 120
47. Case study: 21-year-old has alopecia induced by a tick bite — 122

SECTION V. IMPACT OF LYME DISEASE

48. Complications of tickborne diseases — 127
49. Babesia patients can remain symptomatic for years — 128
50. The risks of pain and fatigue after three weeks of treatment — 130
51. Quality of life for Lyme disease patients can be grim — 132
52. Fatigue can be severe in Lyme disease — 134
53. Does Lyme disease affect your ability to work? — 135
54. Both men and woman can suffer for years after treatment — 137
55. Some Lyme disease patients do well — 138
56. More than half of patients with Lyme neuroborreliosis ill for years — 139
57. The treatment costs of Lyme disease can be significant for patients — 141
58. Lyme disease could cost society billions — 143
59. A second study puts costs at up to $1.3 billion a year — 145

SECTION VI. LIMITATIONS OF LABORATORY TESTS

60. 82 percent of study patients with clinical history of Lyme not tested ... 149
61. Doctors are not testing for Babesia and Anaplasmosis ... 151
62. Testing engorged ticks not reliable ... 153
63. Blood smears unreliable for diagnosing Babesia ... 155
64. Chronic inflammatory demyelinating polyneuropathy case seroconverts to Lyme disease ... 157
65. Lyme disease causes a positive test for mono ... 159
66. Don't eliminate lab-developed test for tickborne illnesses ... 162
67. Seronegative B. miyamotoi ... 164
   Section VII. Challenges of diagnosing the disease ... 166
68. Lyme disease initially diagnosed as juvenile rheumatoid arthritis ... 167
69. Case study: American woman diagnosed after traveling to Columbia ... 169
70. Don't count on a relapsing fever to diagnose B. miyamotoi ... 171
71. Case study: First report of malaria with Lyme disease as a coinfection ... 172
72. Why was the level of hospital diagnoses high during the winter in England? ... 174
73. Babesia difficult to diagnose ... 175
74. Sweats may be helpful in diagnosing Babesia ... 176
75. Signs of Lyme disease may disappear then re-emerge ... 178
76. Up to 40 percent of Lyme disease patients are infected with Babesia ... 179
77. Case study: 70-year-old man ill with babesiosis and Lyme disease ... 180
78. Psychiatric presentations delay Lyme disease diagnosis ... 182
79. Could Chikungunya virus symptoms mimic Lyme disease? ... 184
80. Doctors try to make case for medically unexplained symptoms ... 186
81. Biological explanations might reduce clinicians' empathy ... 188
82. Could a patient diagnosed with fibromyalgia instead have Lyme disease? ... 190
   Section VIII. Conflicts in the medical community ... 192
83. Guidelines should not constrain clinical judgment ... 193
84. Guidelines are too restrictive for doctors in practice ... 195

85. Patients should be informed of conflicting treatment guidelines ... 197
86. Time to designate Lyme disease as a pandemic? ... 198
87. Recommendations ignore chronic manifestations of Lyme disease ... 200
88. Medicine's worst kept secret: Chronic manifestations of Lyme disease exist ... 202
89. The medical community forced out of its comfort zone ... 204
90. 'Fake news' charges do not give professionals credit ... 206
91. Shared decision-making approach to patient-centered medicine ... 208
92. Clinicians urged to tailor therapy based on the patient's response ... 210
93. Doctors should not be impatient or dismissive ... 212
94. CDC takes swift and aggressive action on the Zika outbreak ... 214
95. Center yet to see a Lyme encephalopathy case ... 216
96. One trial and three journal articles, yet the researcher failed to recognize the complications of Lyme disease. ... 218
97. Neither two nor 14 weeks of antibiotics effective in Netherlands trial ... 221

Section IX. Treatment options ... 223

98. ILADS guidelines have been disseminated and implemented ... 224
99. Lingering concerns about the Lyme disease vaccine ... 226
100. Case study: Minnesota traveler contracts B. miyamotoi and B. burgdorferi ... 229
101. Johns Hopkins study supports early retreatment ... 231
102. Antibiotics effective for some but not all neurologic complications ... 233
103. One-time, single dose of doxycycline for a tick bite problem ... 235
104. New combinations of antibiotics effective in culture ... 238
105. Case study: Reversible complete heart block caused by Lyme disease in Canada ... 240
106. Case study: Temporary pacemaker effective in 30-year-old with heart block ... 242
107. Steroid use has been associated with treatment failure ... 244
108. Persistence of infection may drive Lyme disease ... 246
109. Short courses of antibiotics may fail to eradicate the spirochete ... 248

110. Diversity of strains may explain treatment failures	250
111. New drug approaches identified to combat Lyme persister cells	252
112. Antibiotics or life-long immunosuppressive therapy?	255
113. Probiotics may help ward off Clostridium difficile diarrhea	258
114. Case study: Anxious with suicidal thoughts and a history of Lyme disease	260
115. Long diagnostic delays thwart success rate of Lyme treatment	263
116. Hundreds of doctors prescribing longer courses of therapy	265
117. Could monoclonal antibodies prevent Lyme disease?	268
118. Case study: 67-year-old man avoids surgery for arthritis	271
119. Azithromycin gel fails to prevent Lyme disease	274
Section X. Special concerns for children	276
120. Children at greatest risk for being bitten by ticks	277
121. Tick bites: young kids and the elderly have something in in common	279
122. One in three ticks removed from children is engorged	281
123. Only 12 percent of children report always checking for ticks	283
124. Children hospitalized with Lyme disease	285
125. In need of a better understanding of Lyme disease in children	288
126. Case study: 7-year-old with Lyme disease presenting as ADHD	290
127. Case study: 16-year-old with Lyme disease presenting as depression	293
128. Children testing positive for Babesia microti	296
129. Case study: 10-year-old boy with Lyme disease in India	298
Section XI. Education and Prevention	300
130. Half of Connecticut families have had at least one member with a tickborne disease	301
131. How easy is it to pick up a questing tick? Pretty easy.	303
132. How long must a tick be attached to transmit Lyme bacteria?	304
133. Partially fed ticks can reattach to a second host and feed	306
134. Six minutes in your clothes dryer will kill a tick	308
135. Risk of a tick bite higher for pet owners	310
136. Ticks bite during winter months in the South	312
137. Larval ticks a threat with the discovery of B. miyamotoi	313

138. Larval ticks may be a threat to humans after all	315
139. Permethrin-treated clothing causes 'hot foot' effect in ticks	317
140. Lack of awareness of Babesia and Anaplasmosis	320
Section XII. Research and novel approaches	321
141. What could happen to the brain during acute infection?	322
142. T-cell chemokine levels can remain high in Lyme disease	325
143. The brain has exaggerated responses to pain and non-painful stimuli	327
144. New tools might validate brain's exaggerated response to sensory input	330
145. Activated astrocytes could lead to long-term brain injury	332
146. Over-shooting B cell response may contribute to brain pathology	333
147. Slowing down the Lyme disease spirochete	334
148. Persister cells may complicate treatment	336
149. Could dormancy allow Lyme disease to survive antibiotics?	338
150. Does Borrelia DNA persistence cause pain to persist after Lyme 'cure'?	340
References	343
Preview next book.	382
Preview 1: 12-year-old boy suffers cardiac arrest because of Lyme disease	383
Preview 2: Blood donor infects premature infants with Babesia	385
Preview 3: Congenital transmission of babesiosis: two case reports	388
Preview 4: Transfusion-transmitted babesiosis popping up in more states	391
Preview 5: Could autonomic dysfunction lead to pain in Lyme disease?	393
Preview 6: Chronic Lyme disease: Doctors seek answers	395
Preview 7: Children in the Netherlands ill with post-treatment Lyme borreliosis syndrome	397
Acknowledgments	399
Educational videos by Dr. Cameron	400
Lyme disease patient profiles	401
Instagram conversations	402
Facebook conversations	403
Youtube conversations	404

Selected research by Dr. Cameron   406
Links to reading resources   407

ABOUT THE AUTHOR

Dr. Daniel Cameron is an expert in the diagnosis and treatment of Lyme and tickborne diseases. He received both a medical degree and masters degree in epidemiology from the University of Minnesota. He completed a medicine residency at Beth Israel Medical Center and a community and preventive medicine residency at Mt. Sinai Hospital, both in New York, N.Y. His leadership activities include two terms as president of the International Lyme and Associated Diseases Society (ILADS) and at the lead author in the society's two evidence-based treatment guidelines. Dr. Cameron has practiced medicine for more than 30 years in Mt. Kisco, N.Y.

www.DanielCameronMD.com
DCameron@DanielCameronMD.com

facebook.com/danielcameronmd
twitter.com/drdanielcameron
instagram.com/drdanielcameron

COPYRIGHT

No part of this book may be reproduced in any form or by any mechanical or electronic means, including information storage and retrieval systems, without written permission from the author, except for the use of brief quotations in reviews.

For information about permission to reproduce selections from this book, write to DCameron@DanielCameronMD.com.

All Things Lyme Press

Copyright © 2019 by Dr. Daniel Cameron

All rights reserved

MEDICAL DISCLAIMER

The author has cited and interpreted the published literature to provide information on tickborne illnesses. However, as new research and experience broaden our knowledge of tickborne illnesses, and given the possibility of human error, neither the author nor any other party involved in preparing this book warrants information and is not responsible for errors, omissions, or the results obtained from the use of this information. Professionals are advised to independently verify the information and interpretations discussed in these conversations.

This book is not intended as medical advice or guidance for patients. It is no substitute for individual patient assessment by a healthcare professional.

DEDICATIONS

To my wife and family

To my patients

FOREWORD

For more than thirty years, Daniel Cameron, M.D. has practiced medicine with a twist. While he trained in Internal Medicine at Beth Israel Medical Center in Manhattan, he also completed a Community and Preventive Residency from Mt. Sinai Medical Center, also in Manhattan. His public health training from the University of Minnesota and Mt. Sinai Medical Center means while he toils to get patients well, he also teaches them the whys of their illnesses.

When he began to see patients with Lyme disease, he continued to teach patients, but with his Public Health background, he also saw the need to teach a wider audience about the tick-borne disease. To that end, he started a blog he titled: *Lyme disease Science Bloog*. In his blog, Dr. Cameron highlights important research about tick infections, Lyme treatment, testing, medications and other topics related to Lyme disease and co-infections.

As the blogs accumulated, Dr. Cameron thought it a good idea to put the mini-essays into a book which would categorize them by subject matter. But he didn't want just a book of blogs; he wanted the book to have a purpose—actually, he wanted the book to have a life. He envisioned a book which would reach many audiences in many different ways. For those who like the feel of a page, the smell of the ink and love to scratch margin notes, there's the traditional version. For those who want the book on their computer, there's the eBook. You can download it to your desktop; print off the blogs you might want to take to your physician. You can hit a link and go to other sites. Or, load it to your eBook reader and make it portable. In addition to the book, Dr. Cameron has plans for more outreach and discussion on the book's topics.

In short, this book, born of the blog titled, *Lyme Disease Science Blog*, was designed with the needs of the reader in mind. What information might you need as a patient, as a care-giver, as a physician, as an advocate? It's here; and Book Two is in the works.

It was an honor to be asked to help with this project. It was great fun to work with Dr. Cameron. All of those who worked on this book, the videos, the website and other aspects look forward to hearing what you think.

Sue Ferrara, Ph.D.

Editor and contributor

PREFACE

An Ugly Gift From Pandora's Box

The Greek poet, Hesiod, first told the story of Pandora and her box of ills. Created from mud and water by an order from Zeus, *he called this woman Pandora, because all they who dwelt on Olympus gave each a gift, a plague to men who eat bread.*

As the story goes, Pandora (her name means "the all-endowed") *took off the great lid of the jar with her hands and scattered, all these and her thought caused sorrow and mischief to men. Only Hope remained there in an unbreakable home within under the rim of the great jar, and did not fly out at the door; But the rest, countless plagues, wander amongst men; for earth is full of evils, and the sea is full. Of themselves diseases come upon men continually by day and by night, bringing mischief to mortals silently.*[1]

Scientists seem to have opened Pandora's box with the discovery of Lyme disease. We now know ticks were present millions of years ago and that *Borrelia* spirochetes have been infecting humans for thousands of years. We also know, through accidental discovery and direct research, that a single tick can carry multiple infectious agents and thereby transmit more than one disease.

Ticks capable of causing disease have been on the earth for at least 15 million years.

In an accidental discovery, Professor George Poinar, Jr., a palaeoentomologist and parasitologist, identified ticks preserved in a piece of amber estimated to be 15 to 20 million years old. Poinar, from Oregon State University, had acquired the amber while visiting the Dominican Republic 25 years earlier and had just recently examined it with a powerful compound microscope. What he saw was astonishing: tiny fossilized ticks with "ancient bacteria trapped in some of them."

Poinar found spirochete-like cells of *Palaeoborrelia dominicana* in one of four ticks (Amblyomma) preserved in the amber.[2] He could not, however, "attempt to analyze the ancient DNA to confirm whether or not the bacterium is related to modern *Borrelia* because those tests would destroy the specimen," says *Nature* reporter Rachel Nuwer. "But the bacteria's morphology and its location within the tick's alimentary tract indicate that it probably has ties to those notorious pathogens."[3]

Poinar explains that the genome sequencing of the tick's DNA also identified that it "had been infected with the spirochete *Borrelia burgdorferi*, the causative pathogen of Lyme disease."[3] Ticks have been around as long as humans have been alive, says Poinar. "I'm sure that [our human ancestors] suffered from ailments caused by spirochetes carried by ticks."[3]

Tickborne diseases have been infecting humans for thousands of years.

Another accidental discovery dates the Lyme bacterium back at least 5,300 years. Kean and colleagues from McMaster University's Division of Rheumatology in Ontario, Canada, came to that conclusion after examining the body tissues of a 5,300-year-old man found frozen in a glacier pool in the Italian Alps (colloquially referred to as the Iceman, or Otzi).[4]

Lyme disease might not have been discovered were it not for the concern and diligence of two Connecticut mothers.

"In November 1975, a mother from Old Lyme, Conn., informed the State Health Department that 12 children from that small community of 5,000, four of whom lived close together on the same road, had a disease diagnosed as juvenile rheumatoid arthritis (JRA)," writes Dr. Alan Steere and colleagues in a 1977 issue of *Arthritis and Rheumatism*. "During the same month, another mother from the same community reported to the Yale Rheumatology Clinic and to the Health Department that she, her husband, two of their children, and several neighbors all had arthritis. Again most of the children were thought to have JRA."[5]

Based on the mothers' reports, researchers began investigating the cases. Steere and colleagues ultimately describe 51 residents from three contiguous Connecticut communities — 39 children and 12 adults — who had developed an illness characterized by recurrent attacks of asymmetric swelling and pain in a few large joints, especially the knee.

"Several adults described episodic symptoms not necessarily associated with documented arthritis, such as severe headache, periorbital edema, malar or photosensitive maculopapular rash, or swelling of the hands or feet," according to Steere and colleagues. "In addition, seven adults noted profound fatigue and hyperesthesia, sometimes persisting for months after the arthritis had gone."[5]

Recurrences and remission were commonplace among that first cluster of cases. "Recurrences were usually short (median 1 week) and separated by much longer periods of complete remission (median 2.5 months). However, even in an individual patient, both the duration of recurrent attacks (up to 4 months) and the interval between them (up to 23 months) were highly variable and therefore unpredictable," wrote the authors.[5]

In 1982, Dr. Willy Burgdorfer identified the spirochete responsible for causing the sickness among the Connecticut residents. The organism would be named *Borrelia burgdorferi* — after its finder.[6] The illness it caused was called Lyme disease for the community of Old Lyme, where two concerned moms first reported the puzzling rise in similar illnesses among their families and neighbors.

Since the discovery of Lyme disease, an ever-growing number of pathogenic Borrelia species have been identified.

Soon after, in 1992, two additional genospecies — *Borrelia garinii* and *Borrelia afzelii* — were identified in Europe and Japan.[7] In a 2016 issue of *The Lancet Infectious Diseases*, Scott likened the growing number of species to prying open a Pandora's box of spirochetes.[8]

Scott cited the discovery of *Borrelia bissettii* in California,[9] *Borrelia americanum* and *Borrelia andersoni* in the southeastern United States,[10] a *B. bissettii*-like strain in a Florida patient,[11] and *Borrelia mayonii* in Wisconsin.[8] And *Borrelia miyamotoi*, a relapsing fever caused by the *Borrelia* spirochete group has been newly recognized as pathogenic.[12]

In addition to identifying numerous species of *Borrelia*, researchers were finding an ever-increasing number of infectious organisms within the same tick (co-infections), such as *Ehrlichia chaffeensis*, the etiologic agent of human monocytotropic ehrlichiosis (HME) and *Anaplasma phagocytophilum*, which causes human granulocytotropic anaplasmosis (HGA).

Babesia microti was first recognized in Connecticut in 1989, nearly 15 years after the discovery of Lyme disease.[13] In a European study, *Bartonella henselae* was present in 40 percent of ticks.[14] *Bartonella* in the tick is best known as the agent underlying cat scratch fever, acquired through feces of mites on cats.[15]

Multiple illnesses have been described following a tick bite.

Studies indicate chronic neurologic abnormalities were documented in patients one month to 14 years after the onset of Lyme disease and were characterized by memory loss, mood changes, or sleep disturbance.[16]

Lyme encephalopathy patients presented with "mild to moderate cognitive impairment and marked levels of fatigue, pain, and impaired physical functioning," according to Fallon and colleagues from the Department of Psychiatry, College of Physicians and Surgeons, Columbia University.[17]

Patients with Lyme disease have presented with neuropsychiatric symptoms, the authors explain. "A broad range of psychiatric reactions have been associated with Lyme disease including paranoia, dementia, schizophrenia, bipolar disorder, panic attacks, major depression, anorexia nervosa, and obsessive-compulsive disorder."[18]

Thirty-six percent of patients treated with three weeks of doxycycline for an erythema migrans rash suffered from post-treatment Lyme disease syndrome (PTLDS).[19] "At six months, 36 percent of patients reported new-onset fatigue, 20 percent widespread pain, and 45 percent neurocognitive difficulties," according to Aucott and colleagues in 2013 from Johns Hopkins University School of Medicine.

A single tick bite can lead to many hardships.

Fallon and colleagues describe pain reported by patients with Lyme encephalopathy as being "similar to those of post-surgery patients" and their fatigue as "similar to that of patients with multiple sclerosis." Limitations in physical functioning on a quality of life scale were "comparable with those of patients with congestive heart failure."[17] The Klempner trials described the quality of life for patients with PTLD as "more than 0.5 SD [standard deviation] greater than the impairment observed in patients with type 2 diabetes or a recent myocardial infarction."[20]

The impact of Lyme disease on children has rarely been examined. Nevertheless, one study found that 14 percent of 86 children with Lyme disease had neurocognitive symptoms on follow-up. Five of those children developed "behavioral changes, forgetfulness, declining school performance, headache or fatigue and in two cases a partial complex seizure disorder."[21] Children with prior cranial nerve palsy have significantly more behavioral changes (16 percent vs. 2 percent), arthralgia and myalgia (21 percent vs. 5 percent), and memory problems (8 percent vs. 1 percent) an average of four years after treatment compared with controls.[22]

As Hesiod wrote in his book, when Pandora spilled the ills from her box (or if you are a purist, her jar), something remained behind, and that was hope. And the goal of this book, *Lyme Disease takes on Medicine,* is to capitalize on hope. I hope the book fosters conversations between patients and their physicians. I hope practicing physicians, researchers, and the medical community share and discuss their findings in an effort to create better treatments for Lyme disease and other tickborne diseases. And I hope these conversations will ultimately mean patients will soon get better.

ORGANIZATION OF THE BOOK

The book is designed to help the reader understand the challenges medicine faces from Lyme and tickborne illnesses. The conversations here are designed to help building a reader's fluency and understanding, of these conditions.

The 11 sections, are not intended to be read cover-to-cover like a textbook. Rather, you can pick and choose the information you need for when you need it.

Section 1 to 3 identifies the various disease-transmitting ticks; talks about where these ticks can be found; and describes the kinds of tickborne illnesses people can contract—both Lyme and its co-infections.

Section 4 to 5 outlines the growing list of complications, symptoms and hardships associated with tickborne illnesses. Section 6 highlight the difficulties of diagnosing these infections. Section 7 examines conflicts within the medical community since the discovery and rise of tickborne illnesses. Section 8 reviews a few of the treatment options that have been discussed. Section 9 outlines the special concerns needing consideration when children contract these illnesses. Section 10 examines several educational and preventive approaches. Finally, the book finishes with a section devoted to cutting-edge research that draws on material presented in the preceding pages.

The appendices serve as quick references for ticks, the pathogens they carry, and tickborne illnesses.

SECTION 1. WHERE ARE THE TICKS

If you want to know where ticks are lurking, that's an easy one. Pretty much everywhere. They've been reported around the world, including in nearly every state in the continental United States. Ticks prefer rural areas with abundant vegetation, but they also thrive in big-city green spaces. They're spread by humans, deer, dogs, birds, lizards, even hedgehogs. In the discussions that follow, you'll learn about the many species of ticks that carry Lyme and related tickborne diseases and the recent explosion of ticks in unexpected regions of the country.

1

RAPID EXPANSION OF TICKS INTO NEW AREAS OF THE UNITED STATES

On Jan. 18, 2016, *Emerging Infectious Diseases* reported that black-legged ticks, which can transmit Lyme disease, had spread to nearly half of all U.S. counties. According to the report, there had been a 44.7 percent increase in the previous 20 years in the number of counties in the United States that recorded the presence of black-legged ticks.[23]

The ticks had spread to 44 of the 48 continental states. Colorado, Idaho, Montana, New Mexico, and Wyoming were the only states that had not recorded the presence of either the *Ixodes scapularis* (black-legged tick) or *I. pacificus*. The report notes that the "lack of tick records from a county — no records — does not imply that ticks are absent from that county, only that records of ticks having been collected in the county are lacking."[23]

Eisen and other researchers attributed the geographic expansion of ticks, in part, to the movements of mammal hosts and birds.

Given the rapid expansion of ticks into new territories and their ability to carry and transmit not only Lyme disease but a host of other infectious diseases, a decisive response by the Centers for Disease Control and Prevention and other health agencies is sorely needed.

2

TICKS MAY BE IN AREAS WHERE THEY HAVE NOT BEEN SEEN

"The lack of routine systematic surveillance across the continental United States of ticks of public health importance hampers our ability to define their current geographic distributions and to monitor changes in their ranges and densities over time,"[23] says Eisen and colleagues with the Division of Vector-Borne Diseases, Fort Collins, Colo.

If there were more resources to monitor and investigate tick distribution, we might find an even greater number of counties are affected, the researchers point out. Lack of tick records from a county does not mean that ticks are absent from that county, "only that records of ticks having been collected in the county are lacking," they say.

It's increasingly clear that there are ticks and tickborne diseases in the southern United States. "It's important for people to be aware that there may be ticks in areas where they haven't seen them previously so that they can take steps to help protect themselves and their families," Eisen and colleagues says.[24]

3

EVALUATING THE RISK OF TICK BITES AT OUTDOOR EVENTS

A research group in the United Kingdom describes an innovative way to determine the risk of tick bites at an outside event. Researchers asked about 500 participants in a two-day mountain marathon in Scotland to check for ticks on the bodies.[25] Their findings are reported in an *Emerging Infectious Diseases* article, "Use of Mass-Participation Outdoor Events to Assess Human Exposure to Tickborne Pathogens."

The event consisted of two days of long-distance bicycle mountain racing through a tick-infested habitat in Scotland. "Teams of two runners each navigate mountainous terrain, carrying all their equipment for an overnight camp," according to Hall and colleagues from the University of Salford.[25]

To encourage participation in the study, racers were offered a tick-removal service, Hall and colleagues point out.[25] At the end of each day, the racers were given a 1.5-mL tube containing 70 percent ethanol. They were asked to place any ticks found on their bodies into the tube.

Participants submitted more ticks than expected. All 564 ticks removed and submitted were from the species *Ixodes ricinus*, typically seen in Europe. On day 1 of the race, 8.5 percent of individuals were bitten, compared with 13.8 percent on day 2.[25]

The ticks were infected with bacteria typically reported in Europe. Investigators identified *Borrelia afzelii, B. burgdorferi sensu stricto, B. valaisiana, B. garinii,* and *B. miyamotoi.*[25] One of the nymphs was infected with *B. miyamotoi*. The authors did not assess the ticks for co-infections. In other words, some of the tested ticks could have been carrying multiple pathogens.

Larval tick bites were reported in 4 percent and 8.8 percent of participants on day 1 and day 2, respectively. The authors report larval tick bites had been of concern with reports of *B. miyamotoi* infections in *I. ricinus* larvae.

None of the participants contracted a tickborne illness to the investigators' knowledge. The authors presume this was due to the prophylactic removal of the ticks.[25] The study did not follow participants after the event.

Other investigators have identified ticks on human participations in outdoor events:

- Ticks were removed from almost 1,100 visitors to a popular woodland site in southern England during April-October 1996 and 1997.[26]
- 710 tick bites were recorded for 568 soldiers at an outdoor training base in Germany during April-September 2009.[27]
- 22.8 tick bites per 1,000 person-days were recorded in a survey of 931 scouts attending summer camps in Belgium.[28]

The risk of a tick bite in the mountain marathon in Scotland may have been higher than expected because the competitors did not always use clear footpaths and they wore shorts with short-sleeved shirts.

Hall and colleagues provide insight into the risk of tick bites at outdoor events in the U.K. The results "may represent values encountered more widely across Scotland and other parts of the United Kingdom," according to Hall.[25]

It would be reasonable to encourage tick-bite awareness at outdoor events, with organizers possibly offering tick-removal services.

4

"URBAN" TICKS FOUND IN ENGLAND AND CHICAGO

Ticks don't need passports to travel abroad or to vacation at home. Infected ticks have now been found in urban and peri-urban areas of southern England, according to a 2016 paper published in *Ticks and Tick-borne Diseases*.[29]

Questing ticks were collected from grassland, hedges, parks, woodlands, and woodland edges in Salisbury, an urban area located in Wiltshire, England. Ticks were identified at more than half of the 25 sites surveyed, say Hansford and colleagues from Medical Entomology & Zoonoses Ecology, Public Health England, U.K.

Investigators report that 18.1 percent of nymphs carried *Borrelia burgdorferi sensu lato*, 42 percent carried *B. garinii*, and 36 percent carried *B. valaisiana*. Two nymphs tested positive for *B. miyamotoi*, according to Hansford and colleagues.[29]

The repeated presence of male and female nymphs in five sites supported the authors conclusion that urban *Borrelia* transmission cycles may exist in some urban green spaces.

A tick "hot spot" was described at a site based on a high number of ticks and the presence of all stages. At another site, the ticks may have been introduced by a surrounding rural space.[29] The greatest number of ticks were found in the woodland edge.

Both birds and dogs may play a role in transporting ticks into urban habitats. "During the current study, dogs appeared to be walked across a number of green space habitats on the same day, and many survey sites were part of regular walking routes for dogs and their owners. Dogs, therefore, may act as adequate transporters of ticks both into and between urban habitats," explain Hansford and colleagues.[29]

The expansion of infected ticks into urban areas has been a concern in the United States, as well. In a 2007 article titled *"Lyme Disease in Urban Areas, Chicago,"* Jobe and colleagues write, "The high percentage of infected adult ticks identified in this survey highlights the need for physicians in the Chicago area to become familiar with this recommendation, especially considering the high likelihood that nymphal *I. scapularis* ticks are similarly infected."[30]

Whether in the United States or England, ticks are on the move, expanding into more populated regions with recreational spaces frequented by the public.

5

MELTING POT OF TICKBORNE PATHOGENS IN EUROPEAN HEDGEHOGS

*E*uropean hedgehogs are urban dwellers and legally protected in Belgium, making them easy to study. Engorged ticks were collected from hedgehogs in urban and suburban areas at rehabilitating centers in Belgium. In the journal *Parasites & Vectors*, Jahfari and colleagues explain how these European hedgehogs represent a "melting pot" of tickborne pathogens.[31]

The number of ticks per hedgehog ranged from one to 167.[31]

Seventy-one percent of the ticks were infected with at least one pathogen. "Thirty-nine percent of the ticks were infected with more than one pathogen of another genus," according to the authors.[31]

"[The] relatively high prevalence of *B. bavariensis, B. spielmanii, B. afzelii, A. phagocytophilum,* and *R. Helvetica* in engorged ticks suggests that hedgehogs contribute to their enzootic cycles in urban areas," they write.[31]

The European hedgehogs can infect the ticks. The infection rate was higher for *Ixodes ricinus* larvae and nymphs removed from the hedgehogs than for questing *I. ricinus* nymphs and adults collected from the ground.

The authors conclude, "European hedgehogs seem to contribute to the spread and transmission of tickborne pathogens in urban areas."[31]

The authors caution, "Hedgehogs reach up to nine times higher densities in urban areas with parks and gardens than in rural areas, with lowest densities in forests and open grassland fields and agricultural land without cover such as shrubs or dead wood." They add, "Humans are likely to encounter ticks infected with one or several of these pathogens while gardening or recreating in parks."[31]

6

DEER TICKS ALWAYS MIGRATING

Call them wanderers, nomads, or just plain interlopers, but ticks seem to be ever migrating to new areas, but from where? That was the question asked and answered by Khatchikian and colleagues of Penn State's Department of Biology in an article published in 2015 in the journal *Evolution*.[32]

The researchers noted a dramatic increase in the diagnosis of Lyme disease, especially in Pennsylvania which saw a 25% increase between 2013 and 2014. So were cases rising, pondered the researchers, because there were new tick populations? Or was the increase due to an expansion of existing populations?

The answer, the ticks were coming from existing populations and the ticks didn't travel very far. While ticks can hitch rides on deer, birds, white-footed mice and other creatures, the researchers discovered the migration distance of ticks from their established population was less than 62 miles, or 100 kilometers.[32]

"From the point of view of human disease, it doesn't really matter where they come from;" said Khatchikian, "the point is that they're here. But when you start thinking about how to control and prevent infections, it matters to know how easily the vectors of the disease are moving."[32]

The authors end with a grim observation: "The continuous influx of migrants also reduces the chance of local extinctions of tick and pathogen populations and increases the chances of their regional persistence."[32]

The researchers also think homeowners could clear their yards of ticks only to have them return in a week. In an interview Khatchikian said, "If we want to reduce tick populations over the long term, this means we have to start thinking about more sophisticated approaches."[32]

7

BIRDS CARRY TICKS FROM U.S. INTO CANADA, AND FROM CENTRAL AMERICA INTO U.S.

Birds are carrying infected ticks into Canada and the United States. Ogden and colleagues examined the role of migratory birds in the introduction of *Ixodes scapularis* ticks and of *Borrelia burgdorferi* and *Anaplasma phagocytophilum* into Canada.[33]

His team documented the number of ticks crossing the border into Canada during spring 2005 and 2006. They reported that "39,095 northward-migrating land birds were captured at 12 bird observatories. The mean infestation intensity was 1.66 per bird."[33] There were ticks positive for *B. burgdorferi* and *A. phagocytophilum*.

Ogden estimates that "migratory birds disperse 50 million to 175 million *I. scapularis* ticks across Canada each spring, implicating migratory birds as possibly significant in *I. scapularis* range expansion in Canada."[33]

Birds are also carrying ticks into the United States. Cohen describes the phenomenon in "Invasions of Neotropical Ticks and Tick-Borne Pathogens into the United States" in the Dec. 15, 2015, issue of *Applied and Environmental Microbiology*.[34] Most of the ticks on birds were neotropical species with ranges in Central and South America.

Cohen estimates that "anywhere from 4 million to 39 million exotic neotropical ticks are transported to the United States annually on migratory songbirds. Twenty-nine percent of the ticks were positive for infection with Rickettsia species. Only one *Ixodes* genus tick was detected."[34]

Birds can carry ticks for long distances. Cohen writes, "Migratory birds can move hundreds of kilometers, including across the Gulf of Mexico and into the United States, within a short period of time."[34] For example, the 12-gram blackpoll warbler *(Setophaga striata)* can fly up to 2,770 km in three days.[35]

"If such transcontinental movements coincide with attachment and feeding by ticks, avian migration can facilitate the rapid movement of ticks,"[34] according to Ogden, from the National Microbiology Laboratory, Public Health Agency of Canada, St. Hyacinth. "A thrush that had just acquired a tick could potentially transport it up to 1,000 km north in five days."[36]

8

NOVEL WAY TO TRACK TICKS IN CANADA WITH DIGITAL IMAGES

Ticks capable of transmitting Lyme disease have been found in Quebec, Canada, using the traditional specimen-based identification method, where submitted ticks are analyzed by the "gold standard" method using a microscope. But a 2017 study, published in *Parasitology*, demonstrates a different approach of using web-based submissions of digital images or photographs in tracking *Ixodes scapularis* ticks.[37]

"This study demonstrates that image-based tick identification may be an accurate and useful method of detecting ticks for surveillance when images are of suitable quality," explain Koffi and colleagues from the Centre for Foodborne Environmental and Zoonotics Infectious Diseases, Public Health Agency of Canada.[37]

Forty-one veterinary clinics located throughout regions of Quebec submitted digital images of ticks collected from pets using a website for image-based identification by an entomologist, according to Koffi and colleagues.[37]

The investigators acknowledged difficulties in obtaining high-quality images of ticks and instructed veterinarians to orient the tick so the head, dorsal shield, and ventral surface guidelines were visible; that the specimen be in focus, and that a ruler be present for scaling purposes.

Of the 382 tick images submitted online, nearly 75 percent, or 284, were deemed high enough quality to be analyzed. "Of the 284 ticks suitable for image-based species identification, 97 percent were correctly identified,"[37] say the authors.

"Our results showed that images taken of ticks by animal health care professionals (veterinarians and/or animal health technicians) were of a quality suitable to assess the tick species in almost three quarters of cases," says Koffi.[37]

Furthermore, nearly all the 284 tick specimens (254), were in good enough shape to allow researchers to determine the state of engorgement. In fact, in 98 percent of the cases, the digital images accurately identified the state of engorgement. The authors reported that 68 ticks were engorged, 174 were partially engorged, and 12 were not engorged.

"The status of engorgement does not seem to influence the ability of entomologists to perform the image-based identification." The authors note that while the purpose of their study was for surveillance of *I. scapularis* ticks, their web-based tracking tool is also capable of detecting other tick species that may be considered a public health threat.

Koffi and colleagues suggest that citizen-based surveillance methods could be used to detect emerging tick populations and complement traditional surveillance programs.[38]

"If available to the public, an electronic-image-based tick surveillance tool could speed up the monitoring of tick occurrence and activity by removing the need for postage of tick specimens, help reduce the cost of surveillance, and allow rapid feedback to the submitter," the authors conclude.

The Internet provides a great opportunity to gather data on ticks that we have not yet been able to collect. This approach to tick surveillance may be helpful in the United States, where tick records are not always available. As Eisen, from the Division of Vector-Borne Diseases, Fort Collins, points out, "Lack of tick records from a county — "no records" — does not imply that ticks are absent from that county, only that records of ticks having been collected in the county are lacking."[23]

9

ESTABLISHED BLACK-LEGGED TICK POPULATIONS IN TEXAS

*I*nvestigators have identified black-legged ticks (*Ixodes scapularis*) or western black-legged ticks (*Ixodes pacificus*) in 71 of the 254 counties (28 percent) in Texas.[23] Both of those species can transmit Lyme disease.

According to Eisen and colleagues, authors of a 2016 study published in the *Journal of Medical Entomology*,[23] 26 Texas counties (10.2 percent) have established *I. scapularis* populations. And 45 additional counties (17.7 percent) reported *I. scapularis* populations.[23]

Five percent of 1,493 white-tailed deer, tested during the 2001-2015 Texas hunting seasons,[39] were positive for Lyme disease by ELISA, say Adetunji and colleagues from the College of Veterinary Medicine & Biomedical Sciences at Texas A&M University.[39] They add that positive samples in white-tailed deer "correlate with the years in which Texas reported to CDC [its] highest numbers of human Lyme disease."[39]

Only 0.5 percent of the total samples in the Texas study were seroreactive by standardized IgG western immunoblot assay.[40] This should not have come as a surprise given the poor sensitivity of the IgG western blot in actual practice.[17]

Some studies reported removal of black-legged ticks from animals in Texas during the 1980s and 1990s. Adetunji also identified six additional papers published between 2012 and 2016 that report the emergence of Lyme disease in the Texas-Mexico transboundary southern U.S. region.[39]

10

FINDINGS FROM A REAL-TIME ASSAY OF FIVE TICKBORNE PATHOGENS

Five tickborne pathogens were identified in New York and Connecticut using a Multiplex Real-Time Reverse Transcription-PCR Assay. The assay simultaneously detected and differentiated *Anaplasma phagocytophilum, Borrelia burgdorferi, B. miyamotoi, Babesia microti,* and Powassan virus.

Ixodes scapularis ticks were collected in 2015 and 2016 by tick dragging at five sites in Suffolk County, N.Y., at Mansfield in Tolland County, Conn., and at Stamford and Greenwich in Fairfield County, Conn.

As expected, *B. burgdorferi* was the most frequently detected agent in ticks from Suffolk County, with 21 percent of nymphs and 67 percent of adult ticks infected, according to Tokarz and colleagues from the Center for Infection and Immunity, Mailman School of Public Health, Columbia University, New York, N.Y.[41] "The prevalence of *B. burgdorferi* was similar in Connecticut, in 25 percent of nymphs and 62 percent of adult ticks."

The real surprise was the high prevalence of *B. microti,* which was present in 17 percent of nymphs and 30 percent of adults in Suffolk

County, N.Y. In 2014, some 197 babesiosis cases were reported in Suffolk County. The incidence of *B. microti* in Connecticut was lower but still noteworthy at 7 percent of nymphs and 14 percent of adult ticks.

B. miyamotoi was uncommon, being present in 3 percent of both nymphs and adult ticks in Suffolk County, N.Y., and 3 percent of adult ticks in Connecticut.

A. phagocytophilum was less common, present in 7 percent of nymphs and 11 percent of adults in Suffolk County, N.Y., and 7 percent of nymphs and 8 percent of adult ticks in Connecticut.

Powassan virus was even less common, detected in 2 percent of adult ticks in Suffolk County, N.Y., and in 1 percent of adult ticks in Connecticut.

Some ticks had more than one infection.

- One nymph and seven adult ticks (4 percent) were positive for *A. phagocytophilum*, *B. burgdorferi*, and *B. microti* in Suffolk County, N.Y.
- One adult tick was positive for *A. phagocytophilum*, *B. burgdorferi*, and *B. miyamotoi* in Suffolk County.
- One adult tick was positive for *B. burgdorferi*, *B. microti*, and *B. miyamotoi* in Connecticut.

The assay allows for real-time testing for *B. miyamotoi* and Powassan virus in ticks.

The authors stress the consequence of failing to recognize the presence of Babesia as a co-infection with Lyme. "The importance of this finding is underscored by the fact that antibiotics against Lyme disease have no impact on the clinical course of babesiosis," according to Tokarz and colleagues.[41]

11

INFECTED TICKS IN THE SOUTH AS EARLY AS 1991

A recent study on the transmission of *Borrelia burgdorferi* in the Outer Banks of North Carolina highlights the difficulties in determining the actual risk infected ticks present in various regions of the United States. Levine and colleagues, from the College of Veterinary Medicine, North Carolina State University, collected black-legged ticks (*Ixodes scapularis*) at five locations "at varied intervals between 1991 and 2009 and examined for *B. burgdorferi*."[42]

The research team live-trapped mammals including, the "white-footed mouse (*Peromyscus leucopus*), house mouse (*Mus musculus*) marsh rice rat (*Oryzomys palustris*), marsh rabbit (*Sylvilagus palustris*), eastern cottontail (*Sylvilagus floridanus*) and six-lined racerunner (*Cnemidophorus sexlineatus*)". Animal tissues from these species were cultured for spirochetes.

In their 2016 paper, published in the journal *Zoonoses Public Health*, the researchers concluded that ticks and rodents infected with Lyme disease had been questing for 18 years in the Outer Banks. [42]

Yet despite this research, the Outer Banks region has not been designated as a tick-infected area. This lack of designation puts people at risk for getting bitten by ticks carrying Lyme disease.

The researchers noted, "Human cases are primarily being diagnosed in the mountainous, western section of North Carolina." [42] And this is probably not surprising, since the mountains of North Carolina are lush with the kind of vegetation people have come to expect would support ticks.

The Outer Banks, on the other hand, is a 130-mile length of barrier islands off the coast of North Carolina. How did the ticks arrive there?

SECTION II. WHERE ARE THE TICKBORNE DISEASES?

Lyme disease and related tickborne illnesses are infecting people across the United States, but some regions are harder hit than others. Locating Lyme disease hot spots helps put doctors and patients on alert for recognizing symptoms as well as taking preventive measures. The first discussion below proposes an unexpected way to predict where the illness is likely to spike, by mapping the diagnoses of Lyme disease in dogs.

12

USING DOGS TO MAP LYME DISEASE

Our dogs are catching Lyme disease in greater numbers and in a wider geographic region. What does this mean for humans? In mapping the prevalence of the tickborne illness in canines, researchers hope the data may prove useful in predicting areas where human Lyme disease may become a concern.

Researchers mapped Lyme disease in the United States using 11,937,925 *Borrelia burgdorferi* serologic test results from dogs collected within the 48 contiguous states from 2011 to 2015, according to Watson and colleagues from the Department of Mathematical Sciences, Clemson University, Clemson, S.C., in the Journal *PLOSone*.[43] There were 759,103 positive tests for Lyme disease in dogs.

Typically, diagnosis is delayed for dogs with Lyme disease. Based on their review of the literature, the authors summarized several reasons for this:

- "The first signs of clinical disease in dogs are nonspecific, including fever, general malaise, lameness, and swelling of local lymph nodes. These symptoms are likely to be

overlooked by dog owners because they are transient, lasting only a few days."
- "Detecting the later stages of disease requires recognition of pain, however, a standardized protocol for pain assessment in veterinary species is lacking and mainly relies on dog owners to report disease symptoms."
- "The assessment of pain in dogs can be difficult as they cannot self-report and [pain] is often reported by the owner as lethargy, decreased activity, or difficulty getting up, walking, or navigating stairs."
- "It is often not until the dogs exhibit the characteristic shifting leg lameness several months after infection that owners note any abnormalities."[43]

Seropositivity against *B. burgdorferi* was established using the late phase C6 antigen rather than the Centers for Disease Control and Prevention's two-tier surveillance case definition.

The study describes a high prevalence of *B. burgdorferi* antibody in dogs in the 14 states identified in human surveillance: Connecticut, Delaware, Maine, Maryland, Massachusetts, Minnesota, New Hampshire, New Jersey, New York, Pennsylvania, Rhode Island, Vermont, Virginia, and Wisconsin.

The study also describes a high prevalence of *B. burgdorferi* antibody in dogs in other states. "We observed an expansion of this endemic range to include northern California, southeastern Oregon, southwestern Idaho, eastern Colorado, and northern New Mexico," describe Watson and colleagues.[43] "Perhaps most striking is the recognized expansion of seropositive dogs on the northern border of the contiguous U.S. along the Canadian border, including North Dakota and the borders of northern Montana and Idaho."

The study confirms concerns that Lyme disease may be spreading. "The westward expansion of canine *B. burgdorferi* seroprevalence from Minnesota into North Dakota mirrors recent reports that Lyme disease is poised to be a significant human public-health concern in North Dakota," say Watson and colleagues.[43] "Of note is the apparent convergence of *B. burgdorferi* infection of dogs from the northeastern and mid-central United States in the Great Lakes region, encompassing Illinois, Indiana, Kentucky, Ohio, and Michigan.

The author's findings suggest "annual testing of dogs in these states, as well as North Dakota and bordering Canadian provinces, is strongly warranted." According to Watson and colleagues,[43] other regions might benefit from testing dogs. For example, 606 of 57,785 test results reported in South Carolina during 2015 were positive for *B. burgdorferi*.

An annual *B. burgdorferi* seroprevalence study of our dogs could highlight the risks of tickborne illness for dogs and humans.

13

LYME DISEASE CASES JUMP IN THE SOUTHERN UNITED STATES

"The recent confluence of environmental, ecological, sociological, and human demographic factors has created a near 'perfect storm' leading to more ticks in more places throughout North America,"[44] according to the Entomological Society of America Position Statement on Tick-Borne Diseases, published July 29, 2015.

The number of Lyme disease cases has expanded, particularly in the U.S. southern regions. The study, titled "Geographic Expansion of Lyme Disease in the Southeastern United States, 2000–2014," looked at the number of confirmed and probable cases in Virginia and North Carolina during a 14-year period.[45]

Researchers found "a marked increase in Lyme disease cases in Virginia, particularly from 2007 onwards … with development of a new disease cluster in the southern Virginia mountain region." Five counties in North Carolina have been considered endemic for Lyme disease since 2009.[45]

In the coming years, "we may also see expansion into the mountainous areas of neighboring states, such as Kentucky, West Virginia, and Tennessee,"[45] according to Lantos and colleagues from the Division of General Internal Medicine and Division of Pediatric Infectious Diseases, Duke University Medical Center, Durham, N.C.

The study also analyzed public health data from Virginia and North Carolina on more than 11,000 Lyme disease cases reported over a 15-year period. The authors conclude, "The trends in these data paint a clear picture of southward expansion of Lyme disease."

As a result, communities in the southeastern United States once considered non-endemic for Lyme disease will be at risk, the study warns.[45]

14

CASE STUDY: ENTOMOLOGIST ILL AFTER DRAGGING FOR TICKS IN GEORGIA

*D*r. Kerry Clark, an entomologist from the University of North Florida in Jacksonville, had been collecting and studying ticks his entire career before he personally found out the dangers they pose. In 2010, he suddenly became ill after dragging for ticks in Georgia.

Clark began suffering from intermittent pounding headaches, fatigue, odd twitches, and "fuzziness," reports *Discover Magazine*. He tested positive for "traces of *B. burgdorferi* along with another distinct genospecies (a bacterial species separated by divergence of genes), *Borrelia andersoni*, usually found in rabbits." Weeks-long courses of antibiotics would make him feel better, but upon stopping the medication, his symptoms and suffering would return.[46]

In 2013, three years after becoming ill, Clark and colleagues published "Lyme Borreliosis in Human Patients in Florida and Georgia, USA." The study documented PCR and DNA sequence evidence of infection with *Lyme Borrelia* in patients from the southern United States. The report also demonstrates that several *B. burgdorferi* species may be associated with Lyme-disease-like signs and symptoms in southern states.[10]

Clark and colleagues also note that *Borrelia burgdorferi sensu lacto* spirochetes have been identified in birds, rodents, and wild lizards in Florida, South Carolina, and Maryland.[10]

15

LYME DISEASE IN THE SOUTHEAST SINCE 1991

Researchers found that in October 1991, *Borrelia burgdorferi*-infected *Ixodes scapularis* ticks were detected at 50 percent of eight sites on the Outer Banks of North Carolina. "The spirochetes were consistently detected in questing adult ticks at the site in collections made during an 18-year period," explain Levine and colleagues from the College of Veterinary Medicine, North Carolina State University.[42]

The North Carolina investigators went to great lengths to verify the identity of *B. burgdorferi sensu stricto* cases. "The 16 isolates that we sequenced had 98–99 percent homology with *B. burgdorferi sensu stricto*," they say.

B. burgdorferi sensu stricto was also isolated from rodents, including rice rats (*Oryzomys palustris*), white-footed mice (*Peromyscus leucopus*), and marsh rabbits (*Sylvilagus palustris*)."[42]

In their article titled "Stable Transmission of Borrelia Burgdorferi Sensu Stricto on the Outer Banks of North Carolina," the investigators describe strains associated with antibiotic-refractory

Lyme arthritis[47] and with hematogenous dissemination during early Lyme disease.[48]

More than 12 genospecies have been identified in the southeastern United States, explains Levine in his review of three papers.[10,49,50]

The investigators warn readers of the importance of knowing there are *B. burgdorferi* infected *I. scapularis* ticks in that area of the country. They point out that a path through the Outer Banks sanctuary is a routine route for recreational walking, jogging, and bird watching. Such activities pose a potential risk of seasonal human exposure to *B. burgdorferi* infected questing ticks."[42]

16

CULTURE EVIDENCE OF BORRELIA IN THE SOUTHEASTERN U.S. AFTER TREATMENT

*R*udenko and colleagues describe 24 people "who suffered from undefined disorders, had symptoms not typical for Lyme borreliosis, but had undergone antibiotic treatment due to suspicion of having Lyme disease even though they were seronegative."[11]

Three individuals were from North Carolina, 11 from Georgia, and 10 from Florida. Of those 24 people, 71 percent recalled a tick bite, and 50 percent had a lesion resembling that of a tick bite, which ranged in size from a few centimeters in diameter to 9 to 12 centimeters.[11] Their findings were reported in the December 2015 issue of *Clinical Microbiology and Infection*.

Major symptoms included "severe headache, nausea, muscle and joint pain, numbness and tingling sensations in extremities, neck pain, back pain, panic attacks, depression, dizziness, vision problems, sleep problems, and shortness of breath."[11]

The researchers successfully cultivated *Borrelia burgdorferi* and *Borrelia bissettii*-like spirochete from these individuals. This is the "first recovery of live *Borrelia burgdorferi sensu stricto* from residents of southeastern United States," writes Rudenko, and, the "first successful cultivation of live *Borrelia bissettii*-like strain from a resident of North America."[11]

B. bissettii has been examined as a cause of Lyme disease by detection of spirochetes in serum samples in Europe,[51] aortic valve tissue of Lyme borreliosis patients in the Czech Republic,[52] and *B. bissettii*-like DNA detected in north-coastal California.[9]

This strain of *Borrelia* is widely distributed in ticks and wildlife in North America, including in the Southeast. Infection with *B. bissettii* causes Lyme-like symptoms, including flu-like symptoms, arthralgia, weakness, and myalgia.[52]

Rudenko and colleagues concede that typically their subjects would not have been studied because:

- The Southeastern U.S. is not considered endemic for Lyme disease by the Centers for Disease Control and Prevention (CDC).
- Patients were negative by the current CDC surveillance definition.
- They had been treated for an extended time with antibiotics.
- The study was retrospective.
- Patients could have been reinfected.

Nevertheless, the recovery of *B. bissettii*-like spirochetes from individuals in the Southeast highlights the need for further study of tickborne pathogens in that region. Furthermore, culturing live *B. burgdorferi sensu stricto* and *B. bissettii*-like bacterium, even after patients have received extended treatment with doxycycline (some up to nine months), was concerning.

17

LYME DISEASE UNDERREPORTED IN TENNESSEE

The incidence of Lyme disease in Tennessee was 7.7 times higher than that reported to the Tennessee Department of Health from 2000 to 2009, according to a study published in the 2013 Journal of the *American Medical Informatics Association*.[53]

In a second, follow-up study, the incidence of Lyme disease in Tennessee was 19 times higher than that reported to the Tennessee Department of Health.[54] From January 2011 to June 2013, some 1,367 cases of Lyme disease were identified in the BlueCross BlueShield of Tennessee database, but only 74 cases were identified by the Tennessee Department of Health.

The authors note that less than 4 percent of the patients' sampled cases in the BlueCross BlueShield of Tennessee claims database met the national surveillance case definition for Lyme disease.[53]

The authors propose using medically diagnosed cases from a Tennessee-based managed care organization to help bridge gaps in the surveillance system.[53]

18

LYME DISEASE EPIDEMIC IN OHIO

Since 2009, the number of black-legged ticks (*Ixodes scapularis*) exploded in Ohio. In turn, the number of reported Lyme disease cases doubled. Those are the findings of a study conducted by Ohio State University and the Ohio Department of Health.[55]

The authors of the study, published in the June 2014 issue of *Frontiers in Cellular Infection Microbiology*,[55] report a marked increase in deer ticks on mice and the heads of deer during the fall hunting season. The number of I. scapularis found on deer heads increased from 29 in 2010 to 1830 in 2011. Deer ticks were found in 57 of the 88 counties of Ohio in 2012.

The authors confirm the enzootic life cycle of *Borrelia burgdorferi*, the cause of Lyme disease, exists in Ohio based on the discovery of the tick's three active stages (larva, nymph, and adult).

They attribute the increase in ticks and the percentage of *B. burgdorferi*-infected ticks found in Ohio to migrating birds and deer, as well as to human activities.

The number of black-legged ticks and the risks of infection are expected to continue to increase in Ohio, according to Glen Needham, one of the study's authors and professor emeritus of entomology, Ohio State's College of Food, Agricultural, and Environmental Sciences.

However, the case numbers and surveillance map of the Centers for Disease Control and Prevention (CDC) had not reflected the growing risk of Lyme disease in Ohio at the time of the study.

The Ohio study therefore suggests that medical professionals consider Lyme disease and tickborne illnesses even in patients living in states not yet recognized as endemic by the CDC.

SECTION III. CO-INFECTIONS IN TICKS.

The spread of tick-borne illnesses related to Lyme disease, particularly Babesia, further complicates diagnosis and treatment. As it turns out, the same tick infected with Lyme often carries other diseases, too. Lyme and Babesia may look like the same disease with the same symptoms; but it's critical for treating physicians to be able to distinguish between the two because they require different therapies. The antibiotics that fight Lyme disease are useless against Babesia. The following discussions point to the conclusion that one or more co-infections are the rule, not the exception.

19

COINFECTIONS IN TICKS

The spread of tick-borne illnesses related to Lyme disease, particularly Babesia, further complicates diagnosis and treatment. As it turns out, the same tick infected with Lyme often carries other diseases, too. Lyme and Babesia may look like the same disease with the same symptoms; but it's critical for treating physicians to be able to distinguish between the two because they require different therapies. The antibiotics that fight Lyme disease are useless against Babesia. The following discussions point to the conclusion that one or more co-infections are the rule, not the exception.

20

COINFECTIONS OF TICKS ARE THE RULE

Nearly 50 percent of 267 *Ixodes ricinus* female ticks collected in the French Ardennes in 2012 were coinfected, according to a 2016 paper titled "Co-infection of Ticks: The Rule Rather Than the Exception." Among the infected ticks, "45 percent were coinfected and carried up to five different pathogens," according to Moutailler and colleagues from UMR Bipar, Anses, France.

The most prevalent co-infections were *Bartonella henselae* (17.6 percent) and *Rickettsia* of the spotted fever group (16.8 percent), which were mostly *Rickettsia Helvetica*. *Borrelia miyamotoi* was identified in 3 percent of the ticks, while *Babesia* species (*B. divergens*) was uncommon (0.3%).[56]

The authors acknowledge that the co-infections with *B. henselae* remain controversial. "The role of ticks as a vector of *B. henselae* is still heartily debated." An article published in 2010 summarizes the arguments for and against the transmission of *B. henselae* by deer ticks.[57]

Co-infections are also emerging as in the United States:

- Forty percent of patients in the United States with Lyme disease experience concurrent babesiosis.
- Thirteen percent of patients with Lyme disease experience concurrent human granulocytic anaplasmosis (HGA).
- Two-thirds of patients with babesiosis experience concurrent Lyme disease and one-third experience concurrent HGA.[58]

Co-infections create quite the clinical challenge for physicians, since they often must tease out the co-infections by symptoms; tests for many of these infections either don't exist or are unreliable.

BABESIA BECOMES THE NO. 2 TICKBORNE ILLNESS

Babesia has become the second most common tick-borne disease, according to a 2014 trial conducted in Dutchess County, N.Y.[59] Nearly 14 percent of questing nymphal ticks identified in the trial were infected with *Babesia microti*, the cause of babesiosis.

Other tick-borne pathogens were found in the same ticks. Over 29 percent of the ticks were infected with *Borrelia burgdorferi*, the cause of Lyme. Only 8.5 percent of the ticks were infected with human granulocytic anaplasmosis (HGA), the cause of anaplasmosis.

Six percent of questing nymphal ticks were infected with the pathogens that cause both babesiosis and Lyme disease (the most common tick-borne disease). A co-infection of Babesia and Lyme disease can increase the severity and duration of a patient's illness.[60]

Standard antibiotic treatments for Lyme disease, such as doxycycline, amoxicillin, and Zithromax, are not effective for treating Babesia. However, when antiparasitic therapy is added to Zithromax, the combination has been effective for treating Babesia.[60] Other antiparasitic therapies, including Flagyl and Tindamax, also have been used but not described in the literature.

The authors of the study conclude that because co-infection of the two pathogens "can exacerbate symptoms and requires distinct treatment, medical practitioners should be aware of the tendency for *B. microti* and *B. burgdorferi* to co-occur when diagnosing and treating tick-borne illness."

22

BABESIA A GROWING CONCERN FOR BLOOD BANKS

*B*abesiosis, an emerging tick-borne disease caused by the parasite *Babesia microti*, is currently the highest-ranked pathogen transmitted by blood transfusions. The infection can go undetected because infected individuals may be asymptomatic or have only subtle symptoms. But for some people receiving the blood, it can cause chronic, debilitating illness.

Curcio and colleagues express concern over the transmission of Babesia through blood banks because donors are not routinely evaluated for the disease. The Food and Drug Administration (FDA) has not approved and implemented a donor screen for *B. microti*.[61]

"Transfusion transmitted babesiosis has high fatality in transfusion recipients," they say. From 1979 to 2009, some 28 deaths were reported that were attributed to complications from transfusion transmitted babesiosis, they add. Between 2010 and 2014, four deaths associated with transfusion-transmitted babesiosis were reported to the FDA.[61]

Babesia had already been reported in the blood supply. A study in 2012 by Tonnetti and colleagues found that of the 2,150 donations tested in Minnesota between October 2010 and November 2011, 42 donors (2 percent) were positive by IFA.[62]

"It could be expected that the number of tested blood donors in New York State would be higher," explain Curcio and colleagues, "as it represents 37.2 percent of the total number of CDC-reported babesiosis cases."[61]

The authors suggest babesiosis screening for the nearly 5 million recipients of blood transfusions annually in the United States. "The implementation of an FDA-approved screening has the potential to save many lives."

HALF OF PATIENTS WITH BABESIA SYMPTOMATIC FOR MORE THAN THREE MONTHS

"Although not all patients experience severe illness, co-infection [with Babesia] generally results in more intense acute illness and a more prolonged convalescence than accompany either infection alone,"[60] according to Krause and colleagues from the Departments of Pediatrics and Laboratory Medicine, University of Connecticut School of Medicine, Farmington, Conn.

Krause and colleagues note:

- "Thirteen (50 percent) of 26 co-infected patients were symptomatic for three months or longer compared with seven (4 percent) of the 184 patients with Lyme disease alone (P<0.001).
- "Patients co-infected with Lyme disease experienced more symptoms and a more persistent episode of illness than did those (n=10) experiencing babesial infection alone."
- "Circulating spirochetal DNA was detected more than three times as often in co-infected patients as in those with Lyme disease alone (P=0.06)."

Babesia treatment was typically delayed in the cases Krause and colleagues reviewed. "No therapy for babesiosis was administered to any of the subjects; diagnosis generally was delayed," according to Krause.[60]

Babesia patients were typically not immunocompromised. "Although three of the *Babesia*-infected subjects had a history of pre-existing malignancy, no other evidence of immunosuppression was noted in any of the other subjects in the study," according to the authors.[60]

The number of cases of Babesia is on the rise, particularly in the northeastern United States. "Epidemiologic studies have documented that up to 40 percent of patients with Lyme disease experience concurrent babesiosis," according to Diuk-Wasse and colleagues from Columbia University.[58]

Clinicians, therefore, should be particularly cognizant of the disease and consider babesiosis in patients with atypical presentations of Lyme disease or in those who do not respond adequately to treatment.

24

CASE STUDY: SEVEN-YEAR-OLD BOY IN MANITOBA HAS BABESIA

Researchers have identified the first known case of *Babesia microti* in Manitoba, a province of Canada. Authors from the University of Manitoba reported recently in the Canadian *Journal of Infectious Diseases and Medical Microbiology* that a 7-year-old boy, with a complicated medical history that included asplenia (a missing spleen), "acquired an infection with *B. microti* in the summer of 2013 and had not travelled outside of Manitoba."[63]

The boy was successfully treated with six weeks of Atovaquone and Azithromycin.

The University of Manitoba entomologists were not surprised by the case, given that 88 cases of Babesia had been reported in Canada's neighboring U.S. states of Minnesota, North Dakota, and Wisconsin.

The University of Manitoba entomologists were also not surprised given the following evidence:

- Black-legged ticks infected with *B microti* had been collected from six different localities in Manitoba as early as 2010.

- The prevalence of *B. microti* ticks ranged from 1.8 percent to as high as 10 percent in other locations.
- *B. microti* had been detected in the tissues of field-collected rodents at two sites.
- Infected "bird-borne" ticks had been observed in Ontario.

25

B. MIYAMOTOI IS THE LATEST UNDERDIAGNOSED TICKBORNE DISEASE

Potentially important symbionts in ticks have been described by Moutailler and colleagues from UMR Bipar, Anses, France. "In addition to human and animal pathogens, ticks also carry symbionts (interacting species) that may not only play a role in tick biology, but might also interact with pathogens," say the authors.

Borrelia miyamotoi is arguably the best example of a tick-borne symbiont that was eventually recognized as a tick-borne illness. But that recognition took time. "*B. miyamotoi*, despite its global distribution in Lyme disease vectors, remained an incidental finding in field surveys and was thought to be an endosymbiont of Ixodes spp. ticks," according to Telford III and colleagues from Tufts University, Massachusetts, in the journal *Clinical Laboratory Medicine* in 2015.[64] An endosymbiont is an organism which can live inside another organism.

The authors concede that *B. miyamotoi* "is likely a common, underdiagnosed zoonosis wherever Lyme disease is reported."

It would seem reasonable to keep studying whether other symbionts might also contribute to disease. The French authors reported four known or suspected symbionts: *Wolbachia, Spiroplasma, Acinetobacter,* and *Midichloria mitochondrii*. "When adding symbiont prevalences, all ticks were infected by at least one microorganism, and up to eight microorganisms were identified in the same tick," says Moutailler.[56]

26

HIGH FREQUENCY OF B. MIYAMOTOI REPORTED

*K*rause and colleagues likewise point out the importance of monitoring emerging infections, such as B. miyamotoi. "Human B. miyamotoi infection appears to be comparable in frequency to babesiosis or human granulocytic anaplasmosis in some areas and may cause severe disease, including meningoencephalitis,"[12] write Krause and colleagues, from the Yale School of Public Health, in 2015 in *Clinical Microbiological Infection*.

In reporting on a case series that same year, Molloy and colleagues say, "A patient presenting with an acute 'summer fever' and no rash and testing positive by the whole cell antigen serologic test for Lyme disease could actually be infected with *Borrelia burgdorferi*, *B. miyamotoi*, or both."[65]

A clinical diagnosis is tough when we do not know the full spectrum of the disease. The Molloy study only included patients who were treated acutely. The case series definition was limited to patients "who were acutely symptomatic with features or whose laboratory findings were suggestive of a possible tick-borne infection (typically fever, myalgia, flu-like illness, headache, or rash)."[65] Unfortunately, those symptoms, including fever, fatigue, and headaches, are similar to those of other tick-borne diseases and acute viral infections.

In the Molloy case series, *B. miyamotoi* was clinically similar to human anaplasmosis, including abnormal aminotransferase levels (liver tests), leukopenia (low white count), and thrombocytopenia (low platelet count). The blood smear, polymerase chain reaction (PCR), and antibody determination used to diagnose *B. miyamotoi* for the study were not available in most commercial laboratories.

Until reliable tests for *B. miyamotoi* are available, physicians will need to diagnose the disease based on a patient's clinical presentation.

Doxycycline or other tetracyclines, amoxicillin, and cefuroxime were effective based on a few case reports and a series of acute cases. Zithromax was also presumed to be effective. However, the study was not designed to assess the long-term outcomes of patients with *B. miyamotoi*, whether treated acutely or not.

27

PATHOLOGISTS AT MAYO CLINIC IDENTIFY BORRELIA MAYONII FROM SIX PATIENTS

*P*athologists at Mayo Clinic, Rochester, Minn., have described a new *Borrelia burgdorferi sensu lato* genospecies in six patients. The new species, provisionally named *Borrelia mayonii*, was found in the Upper Midwest but may be elsewhere. Symptoms are similar to those seen with an infection from *B. burgdorferi*.

"Five of the six patients with atypical PCR results had presented with fever, four had diffuse or focal rash, three had symptoms suggestive of neurological inclusion, and two were admitted to the hospital. The sixth patient presented with knee pain and swelling."[66] All of the patients were diagnosed with a PCR test.

The investigators used a modified Kelly-Pettenkofer medium to culture the specimens rather than a Barbour-Stoenner-Kelly-H (BSK-H) medium. The positive cultures were further characterized by DNA purification, PCR amplification, sequencing, sequence analysis, and multilocus sequence analysis (MLSA), followed by transmission electron microscopy.[11]

Aucott cautions on the availability of testing for *B. mayonii* in 2016 in

Scientific American. "These tests require physicians to send samples to the Mayo Clinic," he explains, and "that just may not happen."[67]

Until reliable tests become readily available, doctors will need to use clinical judgment.

SECTION IV.
COMPLICATIONS OF TICKBORNE DISEASES

Lyme disease and other tick-borne illnesses might make themselves known with the appearance of a circular rash with a spot in the center (commonly called a bull's eye rash) and a bout of flu-like illness. The patient may recall being bitten by a tick in the recent past. If he or she sees a doctor promptly, antibiotics are prescribed and the infection has the best chance of clearing. But many patients don't connect those early symptoms, or may not have them, and the disease appears to resolve on its own. Too often though, in a month, a year, or several years, the disease reappears with far more serious complications. These include severe arthritis, fatigue, heart disease, neuropathy, depression, and cognitive deficiencies that mimic dementia. Lyme complications often then become chronic, particularly if they're undertreated or treated too late. The next set of discussions look at common and less common complications. The case studies give a clearer picture of how these insidious impairments affect people's lives.

28

LANDMARK STUDY OF CHRONIC NEUROLOGIC LYME DISEASE

Twenty-five years ago, researchers acknowledged the existence of chronic illness due to Lyme disease with a landmark study that described chronic neurologic manifestations. The 1990 study would profoundly impact the future course of research and treatment. Once believed to be caused by an acute, self-limited infection, Lyme disease was beginning to be viewed as a potentially more damaging and debilitating illness.

The study's investigators included Dr. Alan Steere, the physician credited with discovering Lyme disease in 1977. The paper, titled "Chronic Neurologic Manifestations of Lyme Disease," examines 27 patients with chronic manifestations.[16]

The most common symptoms include memory loss, depression, sleep disturbance, irritability, difficulty finding words, spinal or radicular pain, distal paresthesias (tingling sensations), sensory loss, fatigue, headache, hearing loss, tinnitus, and fibromyalgia. Less common symptoms consisted of lower motor neuron weakness, ankle hyporeflexia (below normal or absent reflexes), upper motor neuron weakness, hyperreflexia (overactive reflexes), and increased muscle tone.

The study's description of chronic neurologic Lyme would have a profound influence on the clinical practice of medicine. Investigators reported:

- The time from erythema migrans presentation to chronic nervous system involvement was as short as one month to as long as 14 years.
- Most chronic neurologic Lyme patients presented with mild encephalopathy consisting of memory loss, depression, sleep disturbance, irritability, and difficulty finding words. "They forgot names, missed appointments, or misplaced objects. To compensate they made daily lists. Ten patients had symptoms of depression, and three of them sought psychiatric help or received antidepressant medication. Eight patients had excessive daytime sleepiness and seven had extreme irritability. They became angry over circumstances that previously caused minor annoyance. Finally, five patients had subtle symptoms of a language disturbance, with difficulty finding words."
- Chronic neurologic Lyme could affect whether a patient could work. "Although most patients were able to work, three quit their jobs, three decreased their work hours to part time, and two retired early."
- Seventy percent had polyneuropathy. Eleven had pain in the cervical, thoracic, or lumbosacral area of the spine, usually accompanied by tingling, burning, spasms, or shooting pain in the limb or trunk. Seven had only distal paresthesia with intermittent tingling, or "pins and needles" sensations, in the hands or feet. Sixteen of 19 patients with polyneuropathy had axonal polyneuropathy, with subtle abnormalities or distal motor-nerve or sensory-nerve conduction.
- One patient developed leukoencephalitis six years after antibiotic treatment inclusive of progressive stiffness, moderate weakness and increased tone in the muscles of his

right arm and both legs, and incontinence. This individual improved with intravenous antibiotics.
- Only two of the 27 chronic neurologic Lyme patients had an abnormal spinal tap — one with a pleocytosis of seven cells and the other with an elevated IgG index.
- Most had marked fatigue, which was often a major symptom of their illness.
- Half of the patients had headaches. They had "mild-to-severe, episodic, non-pounding headache in a global, hemicranial, bifrontal temporal, or occipital distribution. They did not have nausea or visual or somatosensory aura."
- Four had mild to moderate unilateral hearing loss, sometimes accompanied by tinnitus.
- Four had symptoms of fibromyalgia.
- Seventeen improved after two weeks of intravenous ceftriaxone, but the "recovery was seldom complete. Six (22%) improved but then relapsed. Four (15%) were no better."

The authors raised several unresolved issues. "The likely reason for relapse is failure to eradicate the spirochete completely with a two-week course of intravenous ceftriaxone therapy. On the other hand, the patients who did not improve may have had irreversible damage to the nervous system, particularly since the response to therapy tended to be worse in patients with longer duration of illness."[16]

The researchers conducted a second study, reproducing the chronic manifestations in a case series of 18 patients who met strict criteria for Lyme encephalopathy.[68] The most common symptoms were memory loss, minor depression, somnolence, headache, irritability, hearing loss/tinnitus, and neuropathy. They also found the chronic patients' recovery differed depending on length of treatment. The 18 Lyme encephalopathy patients were treated twice as long as the chronic neurologic Lyme patients (one month vs. two weeks), and 50 percent had "greatly improved" on follow-up. Two (11 percent) were somewhat improved on follow-up.[68]

Other studies ensued. Fallon and colleagues validated the severity of Lyme disease after four weeks of treatment with intravenous ceftriaxone on standardized measures of fatigue, pain, role function, and cognition.[17]

The chronic neurologic Lyme disease paper has not been without controversy. While some doctors recognize the existence and severity of chronic manifestations of Lyme disease,[69] others remain skeptical.[70]

Regardless, the findings have had a significant impact on both researchers and clinicians. This ground-breaking study has led to the recognition of other chronic manifestations of the disease, including Lyme encephalopathy, [17,68] autonomic dysfunction,[71] neuropsychiatric Lyme disease,[72] post Lyme disease, [73] post Lyme disease syndrome, [74] and post treatment Lyme disease syndrome.[75]

"Chronic Neurologic Manifestations of Lyme Disease" was a breakthrough paper. Prior to the 1990 study, Lyme disease had always been considered an acute, self-limited infection that could be effectively treated with a 10- to 21-day course of antibiotics. This study, however, introduced the potential damage the infection could cause to patients. It has been widely cited as evidence for chronic manifestations of Lyme disease. Since its publication, the paper has been reproduced and cited in the U.S. Library of Medicine's PubMed more than 500 times.

This study opened a new era of hope for Lyme disease patients. The authors are to be congratulated. The paper will no doubt be cited throughout the world for many years to come, shaping future research as we continue to pursue newer and better treatments.

KNOWN COMPLICATIONS OF LYME DISEASE GROWING

The list of complications of Lyme disease continues to grow in the medical literature. It now includes:

- arthritis or recurrent arthralgias, neurocognitive impairment, and neuropathy or myelopathy. In a Massachusetts population-based, retrospective cohort study, 34 percent of patients suffered from those complications for an average of six years after treatment for Lyme disease.[76]
- arthralgias, arthritis, and cardiac or neurologic involvement with or without fatigue. In a Westchester County, N.Y., study, 62 percent of a cohort of 215 consecutively treated Lyme disease patients were found to have suffered from them an average of 3.2 years after treatment.[77]
- memory loss, mood changes, and sleep disturbances. Of 27 chronic Lyme disease patients, 24 presented with a mild encephalopathy that began one month to 14 years after the onset of the disease and was characterized by those symptoms, which also included fatigue, headaches, depression, irritability, and difficulty finding words.[16]
- persistent new-onset fatigue (reported by 36 percent of

patients), widespread pain (20 percent), and neurocognitive difficulties (45 percent)[19]
- Lyme encephalopathy[17,68]
- diffuse axonal peripheral neuropathy[16,78]
- post-Lyme syndrome[71,73]
- postural orthostatic tachycardia syndrome (POTS)[71]
- post-treatment Lyme disease syndrome (PTLDS)[19]

Clearly, it would be reasonable to follow up on Lyme patients for complications of the disease.

30

EYE PROBLEMS FROM LYME AND OTHER TICKBORNE DISEASES ON UPSWING

Ocular complications with Lyme disease are infrequent but can be serious. "Complications such as macular edema, chorioretinitis, and optic neuropathy may be vision threatening and require treatment with corticosteroids as long as the recommended antimicrobial regimen has been instituted, say Sathiamoorthi and colleagues from the Mayo Clinic in *Current Opinion in Ophthalmology*.[79]

The authors describe patients with tick-transmitted diseases presenting with the following ophthalmologic findings:

1. follicular conjunctivitis
2. periorbital edema and mild photophobia
3. Bell's palsy, cranial nerve palsies, and Horner syndrome
4. Argyll Robertson pupil
5. keratitis
6. optic neuritis, papilledema, papillitis, and neuroretinitis
7. myositis of extraocular muscles and dacryoadenitis
8. episcleritis, anterior and posterior scleritis
9. anterior, intermediate, and posterior panuveitis

10. retinal vasculitis, cotton wool spots, and choroiditis
11. retinitis, macular edema, and endophthalmitis

The authors point out that optic neuritis, which is often seen in multiple sclerosis, occurs in Lyme disease as well.

Uveitis can also be a complication of Lyme disease, say Sathiamoorthi and colleagues. "In several cases, spirochetes were detected in vitreous material."[79]

Uveitis is an inflammation of the uvea, which is made up of the iris, ciliary body, and choroid. Anterior, intermediate, and posterior uveitis, along with panuveitis, have been described.[80]

Uveitis can have a wide range of acute and chronic presentations. "Patients with anterior uveitis usually complain of pain, redness, blurred vision, photophobia, and watering," according to Agrawal and colleagues from the Medical Research Foundation, India.[81] "Most of the patients would have had repeated attacks and sought consultation with multiple ophthalmologists, and would have used topical and/or systemic medications on and off."

The true incidence of ocular findings related to Lyme disease remains unknown. One case of uveitis was later dismissed based on a negative serologic test. "At least one of the earlier case reports of Lyme uveitis found spirochetes in vitreous material, yet serological testing was negative for Lyme antibodies,"[79] according to Sathiamoorthi and colleagues.[80]

The authors note that ocular involvement is rare in other tick-borne diseases such as babesiosis, tick-borne relapsing fever, Powassan encephalitis, ehrlichiosis, anaplasmosis, and Colorado tick fever.[79] However, the true prevalence of ocular involvement due to tick-borne illnesses is unknown.

Further, it can be difficult to determine the cause of ocular complaints if there is evidence of more than one tick-borne illness. "One case report[82] describes a patient with optic neuritis and orbital myositis who had serologic evidence of HME [human monocytic ehrlichioisis], *Borrelia burgdorferi,* and Babesia," say Sathiamoorthi and colleagues.

More than one species of ticks is associated with ocular findings, as well. According to the authors, they include *Ornithodoros* genus, *Dermacentor variabilis, Ambylomma americanum, Ixodes scapularis,* and *Dermacentor andersoni.*

The authors conclude that the "degree and frequency of ocular signs and symptoms [vary] widely between the different [tick-borne] diseases." They note, "The ophthalmologist needs to be alert to the possibility of an infectious cause depending on the patient's risk factors. The growing number of Lyme disease cases and other tick-borne diseases ... should heighten clinical suspicion for tick-borne illness."[79]

CASE STUDY: 44-YEAR-OLD HAS HEMIFACIAL SPASM FOR FIVE YEARS

LeWitt and colleagues, from the University of Michigan, describe a case of a 44-year-old woman with hemifacial spasms for five years caused by Lyme disease. She'd had no prior neurological problems when she began experiencing facial twitches. The spasms interfered with speech, eating, and the ability to keep her left eye open.

"Hemifacial spasm (HFS) is a relatively common neuromuscular disorder characterized by spontaneous and irregular involuntary spasms of muscles innervated by the seventh cranial nerve," say LeWitt and colleagues in an article titled "Hemifacial Spasm from Lyme Disease: Antibiotic Treatment Points to Cause."[83]

The woman remained symptomatic for five years and elected to undergo surgical exploration, which "revealed neither contact between the facial nerve and arterial structures, nor any other pathology."

An oral cephalosporin was prescribed for 10 days for a wound infection following surgical exploration of the HFS. "During this treatment and for a few days afterward, HFS completely resolved for the first time since its onset, an experience that led to consideration of an underlying infection," according to the authors.[83]

"Further inquiry determined that five years earlier, the patient had sustained a tick bite which was encircled by a rash and associated with a low-grade fever for one week."[83]

The tick bite preceded the HFS symptoms by about six months.

A lumbar puncture exam and cerebrospinal fluid polymerase chain reaction testing for *Borrelia burgdorferi* revealed the woman was positive for Lyme disease, and she was started on intravenous ceftriaxone (2 grams per day for 56 days).

According to LeWitt and colleagues, "The severity of HFS markedly decreased after this treatment, as did symptoms of chronic fatigue that she had been experiencing. Several years later, the patient resumed botulinum toxin injections for treating her mild symptoms of HFS."[83]

32

LYME-LIKE DISEASE OR BAGGIO-YOSHINARI SYNDROME IN BRAZIL

An article published in the *Brazilian Journal of Microbiology* titled "Brazilian Borreliosis with Special Emphasis on Humans and Horses" examined the growing number of Lyme disease cases in Brazil, where they were referred to as Lyme-like or Baggio-Yoshinari syndrome.

The authors took an in-depth look at Baggio-Yoshinari syndrome and how it compares with Lyme disease found in the United States. Although there are slight differences between the diseases, Baggio-Yoshinari syndrome and Lyme disease shared similarities on many fronts.[84]

Both are neglected in some communities. "Despite the increasing number of suspect cases, this disease is still neglected in Brazil by the medical and veterinary communities," write Basile and colleagues.

Both share similar clinical presentations such as erythema migrans, arthritis, neurological symptoms, and cardiac disease.

Both can be multisystemic. "Baggio-Yoshinari syndrome has been reported to cause neurological, cardiac, ophthalmic, muscle, and joint alterations in humans," they report. Furthermore, it has been associated with a high morbidity "due to the presence of symptom recurrence, severe reactive manifestations such as autoimmunity, and the need for prolonged treatment."[84]

Both can be difficult to diagnose. "The disease is often unrecognized, especially at secondary or tertiary stages when patients do not remember what occurred months or years before the current disease," state Basile and colleagues. "Certainly, many cases of unrecognized chronic neurological or articular disease are in fact cases of Baggio-Yoshinari syndrome not identified and treated at early stage."[84]

Lyme and Baggio-Yoshinari can be associated with pets. The capybaras, a popular Brazilian house pet, is a known reservoir for ticks that cause the Lyme-like disease or Baggio-Yoshinari syndrome.[85] "Pet ownership appears to be a risk factor for human Lyme disease, and this may reflect contact with ticks that have detached from a cat or dog within the household."[85]

Both can have recurrences, "especially if antibiotic treatment is initiated later than three months after infection," according to Basile and colleagues.[84] A Lyme disease patient described by Steere in 1977 had three recurrences.[5]

Both can present with cystic characteristics. "Because motile and spiral spirochetes were never isolated or cultured in Brazil, researchers from LIM-17 assumed that the etiological agent in Brazil was present in cystic form."[84]

Both can suffer from co-infections. "The occurrence of microorganisms with morphological structures similar to *Mycoplasma* spp., *Chlamydia* spp., and non-flagellated spirochetes in the peripheral blood of patients with Baggio-Yoshinari syndrome [were also] seropositive for *B. burgdorferi* sensu lato," according to Basile and colleagues. "Those patients exhibited negative serology for *Mycoplasma* spp. and *Chlamydia* spp."[84]

Finally, diagnosis of both was limited by unreliable serologic testing. There is a low sensitivity and specificity with the ELISA, enzyme immunosorbent assay, or western blotting for *B. burgdorferi*, in part because these tests use antigens from *B. burgdorferi* stricto sensu from the Northern Hemisphere.

"Lyme disease is a condition of extreme importance because it is a zoonosis that causes physical and psychological sequelae in affected individuals," the authors say. "It remains poorly investigated in Brazil, especially in the field of veterinary medicine. Therefore, studies describing the unique aspects of the disease in Brazil and the etiological agents found are needed."[84]

The study of Baggio-Yoshinari syndrome reminds us of the hurdles that patients and doctors in other countries must go through to get tick-borne illnesses addressed.

Update: Oliveira from the Ministry of Health, Brasilia, DF, Brazil was not able confirm Lyme-like borreliosis in Brazil in a letter in the journal Travel Medicine and Infectious Disease.[1] "The interpretations of the results have not followed those recommended by the CDC." writes Oliveira. Only three cases of Lyme-like borreliosis were identified. "This evidence reinforces the hypothesis that Lyme borreliosis does not occur in Brazil." writes Oliveira.

1. de Oliveira SV, Faccini-Martinez AA, Cerutti Junior C. Lack of serological evidence for Lyme-like borreliosis in Brazil. *Travel Med Infect Dis.* 2018.

33

VOCAL CORD PARALYSIS AND LYME DISEASE

In a 2016 case series published in *Voice* titled "Laboratory Evaluation of Vocal Fold Paralysis and Paresis," investigators identified Lyme disease as one of several causes of vocal cord paralysis, a condition that can dramatically impact patients' lives, affecting voice, swallowing, and airway function.[86]

Records for 231 patients with vocal cord paralysis or paresis were reviewed to determine whether testing resulted in a clinically important diagnosis.[86] The authors found the prevalence of syphilis, myasthenia gravis, and Lyme disease were higher than normal in these subjects. Other medically important conditions identified included diabetes and thyroid dysfunction.

Past reports have identified Lyme disease as the cause of vocal cord paralysis. "One case was reported in 1988 [by Schroeter and colleagues[87]], in which a singer was diagnosed with Lyme disease and appropriately treated with doxycycline for three weeks, resulting in improvement in voice quality, return to normal speaking and singing, and normal findings via laryngoscopic examination," state White and colleagues. In 2010, Martzolff and colleagues reported two cases of vocal fold paresis secondary to neuroborreliosis. "Both cases resulted in favorable outcomes after antibiotic treatment."[88]

White and colleagues did not design their case series to test cause. "Although their causal relationship to vocal fold paralysis or paresis has not been investigated or established by this study, the medical importance of having established these diagnoses and instituted treatment is self-evident, and their possible causal association awaits further study."[86]

The more common causes of the disorder remained nonlaryngeal malignancies, iatrogenic injuries, and idiopathic causes, according to White and colleagues. Post-operative dysfunction after retraction, dissection along the recurrent laryngeal nerve, and thoracic malignancy have also been identified as contributing triggers.[86]

Nevertheless, the authors point out the importance of testing vocal cord paralysis patients for Lyme disease, particularly those living in endemic regions. "Because vocal fold paresis secondary to Lyme disease can be treated easily with antibiotics, testing patients with idiopathic vocal fold paresis should be routine, especially in endemic areas or in patients who have traveled to areas in which Lyme disease is endemic,"[86] they say.

"It is important for clinicians, especially tertiary and quaternary providers, to be familiar with the numerous diseases that may present in association with vocal fold paralysis or paresis," say White and colleagues, "and to consider comprehensive diagnostic evaluation to identify serious and treatable causal or associated disorders."[86]

34

LOSS OF LIBIDO AND LYME DISEASE

A cross-sectional pilot study carried out at the Breakspear Neuroscience Department in the United Kingdom reports that 50 percent of 16 serologically positive Lyme disease patients had a loss of libido, compared with 0 percent in 18 control patients ($p<0.001$).[89]

The loss of libido was not associated with either detrusor muscle dysfunction or medications, according to Puri and colleagues from the Department of Medicine, Imperial College London, in a 2014 issue of the *International Neurologic Journal.*

The investigators recommend further study, including the use of a well-validated measure of libido. It would also be helpful to examine whether antibiotic treatment can reverse the loss of libido.

CASE STUDY: 59-YEAR-OLD WITH MITRAL VALVE INVOLVEMENT AND CONDUCTION DISEASE

A 59-year-old man had an oval shaped rash behind his left knee six weeks prior to hospital admission while vacationing in Cape Cod. The rash had been treated with a short course of cephalexin for presumed cellulitis, a medication that has not been effective for Lyme disease.[90]

Three weeks after his vacation, he suffered a syncope event without warning when he got up to use the bathroom. "He found himself on the bathroom floor, not recalling any premonitory symptoms for syncope," according to Patel and colleagues from Brown University's Warren Alpert Medical School.[91] He experienced a sharp reduction in his exercise tolerance over the following weeks.

His evaluation demonstrated severe mitral regurgitation; a dilated left atrium; and a combination of first-degree AV block, atrial flutter, and atrial fibrillation. Endocarditis was ruled out with culture. Ischemic disease was ruled out with right and left cardiac catheterization.[91]

Serologic tests for Lyme disease were positive. Lyme disease was diagnosed and treated successfully with intravenous ceftriaxone followed by 21 days of oral doxycycline. The patient was also treated with oral furosemide for heart failure.

The case illustrates the need to consider Lyme disease in individuals with complex cardiac presentations.

It also raises questions regarding the best treatment for the patient's initial rash. "Cephalexin should not be used to treat early Lyme disease and should be prescribed with caution during the summer months for patients believed to have cellulitis in locations where Lyme disease is endemic," according to Nowakowski and colleagues from Westchester Medical Center, New York.[90]

The patient's cardiac presentation might have been prevented if an antibiotic such as cefuroxime were prescribed because it is effective for both cellulitis and Lyme disease.

CASE STUDY: MYOCARDITIS IN A 15-YEAR-OLD ADOLESCENT

A 15-year-old African-American girl was hospitalized after a three-day history of intermittent retrosternal (behind the breast bone) and epigastric pain, according to a 2016 report in the journal *Pediatric Emergency Care*.[92] The pain was described as "gnawing" and "twisting," without radiation in the sternal and right upper quadrant area. The pain was 9 on a scale of 1 to 10. There was no evidence of costochondritis (inflammation of the rib cage cartilage) or acute cholecystitis (gall bladder problems).

The patient was hospitalized with a presumptive diagnosis of myocarditis. Her initial electrocardiography "indicated normal sinus rhythm but revealed low voltages throughout all leads, widened QRS complex, right axis deviation, and nonspecific intraventricular conduction block," according to Fishe and colleagues from the Department of Pediatrics, Division of Pediatric Emergency Medicine, Johns Hopkins Hospital, Baltimore, Md.

Additional testing revealed a markedly elevated Troponin-I of 15.81 (hospital laboratory criterion for acute myocardial infarction is greater than 0.3 ng/mL), moderately diminished left ventricular systolic shortening, and a trivial pericardial effusion by bedside echocardiogram.

Lyme myocarditis was not diagnosed until the patient developed a second-degree atrioventricular block (Mobitz type 2) and hypotension during empiric treatment with 1 g/kg intravenous immune globulin (IVIG).

She was empirically started on doxycycline, along with milrinone infusion for afterload reduction and intravenous furosemide for pulmonary edema.

Her EKG changed to first-degree heart block by hospital day 2 and resolved completely on day 3. The authors note that a Cochrane review found insufficient evidence to support IVIG use in acute myocarditis.[93]

Her Lyme disease was subsequently confirmed with serologic tests. Lyme enzyme-linked immunosorbent assay (ELISA) and immunoglobulin M (IgM) of 0.87 (reference range, 0.00 to 0.79) were positive.

The girl recovered and was discharged home on hospital day 7 on oral furosemide, enalapril, and doxycycline, according to Fishe and colleagues.

"It is important to explain all results that are found as part of the diagnostic work-up," the authors conclude. Furthermore, "in patients with Lyme disease who complain of cardiopulmonary symptoms, clinicians should have a low threshold for obtaining an EKG to evaluate for Lyme carditis."[92]

37

POSTMORTEM FINDINGS EXPLORED FOR FIVE PATIENTS WHO DIED OF LYME CARDITIS

Researchers describe an autopsy study of five patients who suffered sudden cardiac death and were found on postmortem to have Lyme carditis. The cases are discussed in a 2016 article titled "Cardiac Tropism of Borrelia burgdorferi: An Autopsy Study of Sudden Cardiac Death Associated with Lyme Carditis," published in *The American Journal of Pathology*.

Two patients were diagnosed during unexplained-death investigations at the Centers for Disease Control and Prevention (CDC). Lyme disease was suspected in two of the other cases by cardiac pathology at a tissue bank transplant service. Muehlenbachs and colleagues reassured readers that cardiac tissue was not transplanted.[94]

Autopsies uncovered several findings:

Spirochetes were present in the hearts of all five subjects. When using immunohistochemistry (IHC), spirochetes were found "within the myocardial interstitial infiltrates, in the subendocardium, and occasionally in pericardial tissue in association with lymphohistiocytic infiltrates," Muehlenbachs and colleagues say. "Rare spirochetes were seen in the leptomeninges of two cases by immunohistochemistry."

All five subjects lived in Lyme-endemic areas. Patients resided in states with a high or moderate incidence of Lyme disease, including Indiana, Massachusetts, New Hampshire (with recent travel to Connecticut), and New York.

All five subjects reportedly engaged in outdoor activities. "Two patients had known exposure to ticks, and one patient reported a recent bite," the authors say.

None of the five subjects met the CDC surveillance case definition for Lyme carditis. That definition includes recurrent, brief attacks (weeks or months) of objective joint swelling in one or several joints, lymphocytic meningitis, cranial neuritis, radiculoneuropathy, encephalomyelitis, acute onset of high-grade (second- or third-degree) atrioventricular conduction defects, and myocarditis.

Only one of the five subjects underwent serologic screening for Lyme disease, and the results were negative.

All five subjects were symptomatic prior to death. "A prodrome was reported for each of the patients that included the following: nonspecific viral-like illness, malaise, shortness of breath, and anxiety," according to Muehlenbachs and colleagues. Three of these patients had joint pain. A prodrome is an early sign that one is getting sick.

"No dermatologic lesion was documented or reported for any of the patients, although one patient was evaluated in an emergency department one month before death for an arm lesion," the authors say. The lesion was "diagnosed as a possible spider bite from which methicillin-resistant Staphylococcus aureus was isolated in culture."

All five subjects were seropositive postmortem according to the CDC's two-tier criteria. "One sample met both IgM and IgG western blot (WB) criteria, with two of the three IgM bands and 6 of the 10 IgG bands reactive. The four remaining samples were positive by IgM WB criteria only, although three were nearly IgG positive with 4 of the 10 bands reactive," say Muehlenbachs and colleagues.

Underlying cardiac disease may have played a role in three of the five cases of sudden cardiac death associated with Lyme disease. Muehlenbachs and colleagues point out that there was significant underlying heart disease present in two patients, and an additional patient had moderate atherosclerosis discovered at autopsy.

Physiological cardiac stress was considered a potential factor in two of the five subjects. "In the other two patients, who were otherwise healthy, a degree of physiological cardiac stress likely was present: the woman had given birth six months previously and the man was a physically active outdoor enthusiast," according to Muehlenbachs and colleagues.

These pathologic findings provide insight into the possible cause of sudden cardiac death associated with Lyme disease. "The findings support the proposed disease mechanism of spirochete cardiac tropism during early disease dissemination, the infiltration of cardiac tissue by inflammatory cells, and involvement of the conduction system, which likely mediates sudden cardiac death,"[94] the authors say.

"Early diagnosis and prompt treatment for Lyme carditis can be life-saving," they add. "Health care professionals should evaluate all patients with suspected Lyme disease for cardiac signs and symptoms, and obtain an electrocardiogram promptly if carditis is suspected." Furthermore, "Diagnosis is based on clinical suspicion and serologic testing, with the caveat that serology testing may be falsely negative in a patient with recent illness onset."[94]

38

CASE STUDY: DIPLOPIA AND HEART BLOCK IN EARLY-DISSEMINATED LYME DISEASE

A 49-year-old man from Minnesota "met criteria for early disseminated Lyme disease with multiple erythema migrans lesions and evidence of cardiac and neurologic involvement," according to Blackwell and colleagues from the Department of General Internal Medicine, Mayo Clinic.[95]

The patient's exposure included a tick removed from his outdoor cat one month prior to evaluation. His laboratory tests were positive on both a Lyme enzyme-linked immunosorbent assay screening and confirmatory western blot with 3 IgM bands: p41, p39, and p23. His electrocardiography revealed new second-degree Mobitz type I heart block. He was admitted for additional work-up and monitoring.

A magnetic resonance imaging (MRI) was arranged within 24 hours of admission. The image "revealed abnormal enhancement of the bilateral oculomotor nerves, left trigeminal nerve, and probable left abducens nerve, consistent with disseminated Lyme disease," according to the authors.[95]

His rash, heart block, fatigue, and myalgia improved quickly on initiation of a four-week course of intravenous ceftriaxone.

It is unclear if the heart block, diplopia, hospitalization, and four weeks of intravenous ceftriaxone could have been prevented if the 49-year-old had been treated for Lyme disease a month earlier at the onset of the rash. The case report did not discuss whether the antibiotics resolved the diplopia.

CASE STUDY: PHYSICIAN WITH LYME DISEASE THRIVES AFTER HEART TRANSPLANT

Dr. Neil Spector, a leading researcher and oncologist at Duke University Medical Center, Durham, North Carolina, has become a leader in the Lyme disease community. In his memoir, *Gone in a Heartbeat: A Physician's Search for True Healing*, Spector chronicles his battle with debilitating and at times life-threatening cardiac problems caused by undiagnosed Lyme carditis.[96]

Despite his standing within the medical community, physicians and colleagues minimized his complaints, attributing them to stress. Years passed, and his health deteriorated. Eventually he was faced with having to undergo a heart transplant.

Following are excerpted quotes from an interview with Peoples Pharmacy that aired August 15, 2015:[97]

The Misdiagnosis

I was misdiagnosed for four years, mostly because I didn't have the classic symptoms of Lyme disease, which we think of as having the bull's-eye rash, flu-like symptoms … arthritis, fever. I didn't have any of those symptoms. I presented with cardiac symptoms. That's not the common presentation, so my doctors completely misdiagnosed the disease.

I was told that I had stress. I think a lot of people with Lyme are told that their symptoms are not related to anything but stress.

The Misconceptions

Fifty percent of the people don't have the classic bull's-eye rash … and many people don't even have the classic flu-like illness. And if you're in an area where your doctors deny that Lyme disease even exists, then you're really in trouble.

The bacteria that causes Lyme disease is rather unique in that it finds hidden places where antibiotics are not that effective. So, it gets into your connective tissue, around your joints … in your heart … connective tissue in the brain. And those are sanctuaries where antibiotic drug levels generally don't achieve … therapeutic levels. Once it gets into those privileged sanctuaries, it becomes much more difficult to treat.

The Controversy

There's this friction between physicians in the community, who are seeing the real Lyme disease cases and people suffering, and people in academic centers in the Northeast who are saying, "Ah, those doctors in the community are overtreating, they're quacks, they're preying off this fear of chronic Lyme disease."

The Research

I think the amount that the National Institutes of Health spends on Lyme disease is a drop in the bucket compared to what it should be.

CASE STUDY: 18-YEAR-OLD MAN DIES FROM LYME CARDITIS

In the summer of 2013, an 18-year-old man from Poughkeepsie, N.Y., died suddenly after suffering from flu-like symptoms for nearly three weeks. Initial reports suggested he had died from complications of the Powassan virus, a rare but potentially fatal illness transmitted by ticks. However, the young man had, in fact, died from Lyme carditis, reports a paper published in the March 2015 issue of *Cardiovascular Pathologist*.[98]

He had participated in an outdoor camp in a tick-endemic region. Additionally, he lived in Dutchess County, N.Y., an area that's endemic for Lyme disease and where up to 50 percent of adult deer ticks are infected with the Lyme organism. Yet he was neither diagnosed nor treated for Lyme disease.

According to the autopsy, PCR (polymerase chain reaction) and immunohistochemistry staining found *Borrelia* spirochetes present in the patient's liver, heart, lung, and brain tissues. The ELISA and Western blot IgM tests were positive for *Borrelia burgdorferi*.

"The findings support *B. burgdorferi* as the causative agent for his fulminant carditis and that the patient suffered fatal Lyme carditis," the authors write.[98]

It is unfortunate that the focus on a potential Powassan virus overshadowed the risk of Lyme disease. It would have been reasonable for the doctors to have treated for Lyme disease while waiting for the Powassan serologic tests.

41

CASE STUDY: 79-YEAR-OLD WITH LYME MENINGITIS, MANIFESTING AS PARKINSON'S DISEASE

A 79-year-old man had symptoms initially attributed to idiopathic Parkinson's disease but later found to be due to Lyme meningitis. His case is described by Patel and colleagues in an abstract published in *Critical Care Medicine* titled "Atypical Lyme Meningitis with Parkinson Disease-Like Manifestations."[99]

The patient experienced two months of rapidly progressing weakness and persistent headache, explain Patel and colleagues. "He developed a shuffling, wide-based gait without rigidity, predominantly left-sided bradykinesia, marked intention tremor, postural tremor, hypomimia, hypophonia, and positive Romberg test."[99]

He had a history of a follicular lymphoma that was in remission. The authors ruled out cancer with a computed tomography (CT) and CT angiogram of the head and paraneoplastic work-up.

Lyme meningitis was diagnosed based upon the following:

- cerebral spinal fluid analysis with six white blood cells per cubic mm and 95 percent lymphocytes
- positive Lyme serology (titer 2.57 LIV)

- history of tick exposure as an avid hunter
- multiple tick bites after each outing
- absence of another infection

Treatment was successful with IV ceftazidime 1 gram every eight hours for two days followed by a four-week course of ceftriaxone 2 grams IV. "Within 4 weeks of therapy, his headache had resolved and he walked independently without difficulty."[99]

Parkinson's disease is a group of heterogeneous, degenerative, neurological disorders, typically treated with levodopa-carbidopa. Parkinsonism plus syndrome differs from the classic idiopathic Parkinson's disease in certain associated clinical features, poor response to levodopa, distinctive pathological characteristics, and poor prognosis," according to Mitra and colleagues.[100]

The wide range of Parkinsonian syndromes include idiopathic Parkinson's disease, progressive supranuclear palsy, multiple system atrophy, corticobasal degeneration, and vascular Parkinsonism, according to Litvan and colleagues from the University of California.[101]

Patel and colleagues conclude, "Lyme meningitis merits consideration in endemic areas in cases of subacute onset of Parkinsonism of unknown etiology, as it may be fully reversible with antibiotic therapy."[99]

42

CASE STUDY: LYME DISEASE WITH SUBACUTE PARKINSONISM AND ABNORMAL DAT SCANS

Medicine is always on the lookout for reversible causes of common illnesses. Doctors in France describe two cases with patients "who developed reversible subacute parkinsonism due to Lyme basal ganglia ischemic or inflammatory lesions" in the *Journal of Neurology*.[102] The two cases resolved with 21 days of intravenous ceftriaxone for one patient and 42 days for the other.

A 55-year-old patient presented with a two-month history of chronic neck pain and progressive marked asthenia. "Clinical examination revealed a dysarthria which disappeared in less than one hour, a left upper limb cerebellar ataxia, and a bilateral asymmetric mild akinetohypertonic parkinsonism," according to Pisché and colleagues from the Department of Neurology, CHRU Strasbourg, Strasbourg Cedex, France.[102]

A 63-year-old woman developed a rapidly deteriorating, severe walking disorder over six months. "Clinical examination revealed lower limbs weakness, increased reflexes, bilateral extensor plantar, and dysuria, as well as a left akineto-hypertonic syndrome," according to Pisché and colleagues. Facial palsies were also described.[102]

Brain MRI's showed vascular demyelination consistent with that seen in inflammatory, infectious, drug-induced, or paraneoplastic vasculitis conditions.

Both Lyme disease patients presented with abnormal DaTscans, demonstrating "apresynaptic dopaminergic denervation, which has been associated with striatal ischemic lesions due to Lyme probable vasculitis," according to Pisché and colleagues.[102]

DaTscans have been used in Parkinson's disease to allow physicians to provide accurate clinical management of the patient and prevent unnecessary medications and procedures, according to Seifer and colleagues from Florida Atlantic University.[103]

Both patients were diagnosed and treated successfully for Lyme disease. They "developed and fulfilled the diagnostic criteria for neuroborreliosis: no past history of neuroborreliosis, positive anti-BB antibody index, favorable outcome of neurological signs after specific antibiotic treatment, and absence of other diagnosis," according to Pisché and colleagues[102]

The first patient resolved the subacute parkinsonism with a 21-day course of 2 g per day of ceftriaxone without the need for dopaminergic treatment. The second patient required a second 21-day course of ceftriaxone, along with three months of corticosteroid therapy (60 mg per day) and Ldopa/carbidopa (300 mg per day).[102]

"These two cases demonstrate that an acute or subacute parkinsonism may be a complication of Lyme disease," according to Pisché and colleagues[102]

The authors advise that Lyme disease be discussed in endemic areas with basal ganglia MRI lesions. "In front of an acute or subacute parkinsonism, especially in endemic region, neuroborreliosis should be discussed in case of associated headache, multisystemic neurological signs, or MRI basal ganglia vasculitis or inflammatory sign."[102]

They caution, "Lyme blood or CSF serology should not be asked for, even in [an] endemic region, in case of progressive parkinsonism without any basal ganglia MRI lesions."[102]

43

STROKE MANIFESTATIONS OF LYME DISEASE

Strokes should be added to the list of manifestations of Lyme disease based on a 2007 systematic review published in *Frontiers in Neurology*.[104] The authors identified 88 patients in the literature presenting with cerebrovascular course of Lyme neuroborreliosis.

More than half of the cases were from three countries: "16 (25.4 percent) from Germany, 9 (14.3 percent) from Switzerland, and 8 (12.7 percent) from France," note Garkowski and colleagues from the Department of Radiology, Medical University of Białystok, Białystok, Poland.[104] Five (8 percent) were from the United States.

Many of the stroke patients were young. More than half were younger than 50. There were 15 pediatric cases. The youngest was 4 years old (median age 46 with a range of 4 to 77 years). Fifty-four percent were male.

"The most common cerebrovascular manifestation of Lyme neuroborreliosis was ischemic stroke (76.1 percent), followed by TIA (11.4 percent)," according to Garkowski and colleagues.[104] They add, "The posterior circulation was affected alone in 37.8 percent of patients, the anterior circulation in 24.4 percent of patients, and in 37.8 percent of cases, posterior and anterior circulations were affected simultaneously."

Three-quarters of patients had a complete response, which the authors define as "a complete response to antibiotic treatment with halted progression of the disease and no recurrence of cerebral ischemia or recuperation from neurological deficits."

The mortality rate was 4.7 percent. The outcome for the remaining 20 percent was incomplete or incomplete with residual neurologic deficit.

The author suggests prompt evaluation of prodromal syndromes. "The lack of awareness of this manifestation of LNB [Lyme neuroborreliosis] might result in the delay of diagnosis, which might lead even to the patient's death," according to Garkowski and colleagues.[104] They add, "Several weeks/months before stroke onset, prodromal symptoms suggesting LNB, such as meningitis, cranial neuritis, or radiculoneuritis, should prompt extensive diagnostics including CSF [cerebrospinal fluid] examination."

44

CASE STUDY: 43-YEAR-OLD HAS COGNITIVE ISSUES FOLLOWING A STROKE

A 2015 study by Almoussa and colleagues in *Case Reports Neurologic Medicine* serves as a reminder that an infection from *Borrelia burgdorferi* can trigger cognitive impairments. The authors describe a 43-year-old patient from Germany who suffered a stroke due to Lyme disease and continued to have cognitive issues despite treatment.[105]

The patient was previously healthy with no cardiovascular risk factors, but he had a two-week history of malaise, headache, and amnestic cognitive impairment. He recalled having a tick bite four months earlier in the Netherlands but not an erythema migrans rash. The patient presented with a discrete left-sided hemiparesis. He was fully oriented but showed massively slowed movements, marked short-term memory loss, and a mildly stiff neck, but he was oriented to time, place, and person.

His MRI was consistent with a right thalamic infarct. His spinal tap revealed meningitis with an elevated Bb antibody index and the presence of immunoblot antigens of *B. burgdorferi*.

After a three-week course of intravenous ceftriaxone at a dosage of 2 g daily, the patient's left-sided hemiparesis and psychomotor impairment quickly normalized. The signal abnormalities on cranial MRI scans also resolved.

However, the patient's cognitive impairment did not normalize. "Unfortunately, the cognitive amnestic impairment did not improve and the patient was discharged to a stationary cognitive rehabilitation therapy," the authors report.[105] "Despite the quick radiological and clinical response to antibiotic therapy, a mild short-term memory loss was still persistent at the follow-up visit two months later."

Intravenous ceftriaxone was stopped at three weeks based on the European Federation of the Neurological Societies (EFNS) guidelines. The authors did not examine the perennial question of whether additional antibiotics might have resolved cognitive problems after a stroke.

CASE STUDY: KRIS KRISTOFFERSON'S DEMENTIA WAS UNDIAGNOSED LYME DISEASE

For several years, legendary singer and songwriter Kris Kristofferson was believed to be suffering from Alzheimer's disease or dementia. However, the musician's memory problems were later identified as undiagnosed, untreated Lyme disease.

According to a story in the June 6, 2016, issue of *Rolling Stone*, doctors had believed the 79-year-old singer's "increasingly debilitating memory loss was due to either Alzheimer's, or due to dementia brought on by blows to the head from the boxing, football and rugby of his teens and early twenties." He reportedly could not remember what he was doing from one moment to the next, the magazine reports.[106]

For 10 years, Kristofferson was treated unsuccessfully for Alzheimer's disease. After he was diagnosed and treated for Lyme disease, his life changed. Kristofferson's wife, Lisa, explained that once her husband stopped taking medication for Alzheimer's and depression; and underwent three weeks of treatment for Lyme disease; his memory and mood changes were shocking. "All of a sudden he was back," she says. "There are still bad days, but some days he's perfectly normal and it's easy to forget that he is even battling anything," she told *Rolling Stone*.

46

CASE STUDY: TWO MORE PATIENTS WITH REVERSIBLE LYME DISEASE DEMENTIA

The high-profile news that Kris Kristofferson had been suffering from treatable Lyme disease dementia, not Alzheimer's disease, reminds us of the need to consider Lyme disease more often as a possible cause of dementia.[106]

The Washington Post reported June 6, 2016, on an 81-year-old retired case officer from the Defense Intelligence Agency who, after surviving leukemia, was told he had dementia.[107] He was later diagnosed with Lyme meningoencephalitis.

Doctors had believed the man was suffering from "a rapidly progressive and fatal dementia, possibly a particularly aggressive form of Alzheimer's disease," writes *Washington Post* reporter Sandra Boodman.[107] He became "moody, confused, and delusional–even childish–a jarring contrast with the even-keeled, highly competent person he had been." He developed tremors in his arms, had trouble walking, and became incontinent.

After testing positive for Lyme disease, the man began antibiotic treatment and ultimately made a full recovery.

Another 2016 case report was discussed in the *Journal of the*

Neurological Sciences. A 75-year-old woman had been admitted to a hospital in Austria with increasing malaise, abdominal discomfort, nausea, and constipation. She presented with a 10-month cognitive decline, "low mood," and loss of orientation to time, as well as impaired attention, concentration, and short-term memory.[108]

Her examination revealed a marked slowing of speech and movement with word-finding difficulties; rigor and bradykinesia in the right arm; unsteady, broad-based, short-stepped gait with forward flexed trunk posture; and mildly painful nuchal rigidity, but no photophobia.

The MiniMental State Examination (MMSE) score was 20 (out of 30) points. An MRI (magnetic resonance imaging) of the brain showed mild periventricular white matter changes and slight widening of the lateral ventricles, indicating the differential of possible early normal pressure hydrocephalus (NPH).

Several diagnoses were possible beyond dementia and NPH. The woman had long-standing drug treatment for depression, anxiety, headaches, and musculoskeletal pain, as well as mild head trauma from a motor vehicle accident 33 months prior to admission.

Lyme disease was diagnosed based on an abnormal spinal tap. Her cerebrospinal fluid (CSF) evaluation revealed what the authors concluded was Lyme neuroborreliosis. The CSF had a "predominantly lymphocytic pleocytosis, elevated protein, oligoclonal bands and a highly positive CSF/serum Bb-specific IgG index."

"Late Lyme neuroborreliosis was diagnosed according to current European guidelines," point out Topakian and colleagues.[108] The woman improved with three weeks of intravenous ceftriaxone. After completion of that antibiotic therapy, her MMSE score was 28 out of 30 and all neurologic signs resolved. The repeat CSF was clear, and the patient's health had remained well on 15-month follow-up.

Such stories and case reports remind us of the importance of considering Lyme disease as another cause of dementia, and one that's reversible.

CASE STUDY: 21-YEAR-OLD HAS ALOPECIA INDUCED BY A TICK BITE

In a recent issue of the *American Journal of Dermatopathology*, Lynch and colleagues report the case of a 21-year-old man who suffered hair loss (alopecia) following a tick bite to the scalp.[109] The man presented with non-scarring alopecia and a pattern of hair loss similar to alopecia-areata, also known as spot baldness.

Tick-bite-induced non-scarring alopecia typically presents as patches, often described as "motheaten," or nodular, blood-crusted lesions. According to the authors, symptoms include pain, pruritus (itching), or swelling. "There is usually a history of tick bite to affected areas, but lack of patient-reported tick attachment does not rule out this diagnosis."[109]

The patient's non-scarring tick-borne alopecia was complicated by external trauma, including hair pulling and lichen simplex chronicus, a condition of thick, leathery, brownish skin caused by chronic itching and scratching.

Researchers suggest the alopecia results from the body's immune response to tick bite. "Tick-bite alopecia is a reported phenomenon that is thought to be caused by a robust host response to tick-injected saliva containing anticoagulant and anti-inflammatory and immunomodulatory chemicals," explain Lynch and colleagues.

"To the authors' knowledge, this is the fifth report of nonscarring tick-bite alopecia in the literature and the first in an adult patient," they write.[109]

There is good news for patients with non-scarring tick-borne alopecia. "Because few hair follicles are truly destroyed in this form of tick-bite alopecia, hair regrowth is commonly observed, usually within 3 months;[110-112] however, alopecia has been reported to persist for 5 years after healing of local reaction to tick bites," according to a series of four papers cited by Lynch and colleagues.[113]

A scarring form of tick-bite alopecia has been described in Europe. "Tick-borne lymphadenopathy syndrome, classically transmitted by ticks of the genus *Dermacentor* and caused by *Rickettsia slovaca* infection, is an emerging entity typically seen in Europe," according to Lynch and colleagues. "Doxycycline remains the treatment of choice."[109]

Generalized hair loss also has been described in Lyme disease patients.[114] "Diffuse alopecia occurred within three months after the outbreak of disease in 3 out of 23 (13 percent) patients with Lyme meningitis and in 40 out of 71 (56.3 percent) patients with tick-borne encephalitis," according to Cimperman and colleagues from the University Medical Centre, Ljubljana, Slovenia. "The mean duration of alopecia was 2 to 3 months and alopecia was reversible in all patients."[114]

Scarring and nonscarring alopecia have a number of causes, including autoimmune conditions such as lupus, diabetes, and fibromyalgia.[115] Moreover, medications used to treat systemic autoimmune disease and fibromyalgia have also been associated with alopecia.

Hair loss can impair the quality of life of patients with systemic disease. "Patients in remission from their global systemic disease are often left with alopecia, which significantly impairs their self-esteem and interferes with their personal and professional lives," according to Moghadam-Kia and colleagues from the University of Pittsburgh Medical Center. "This situation is often not adequately recognized, and withdrawal from social and work functions often leads to or augments long-standing depression in the patient."[115]

SECTION V. IMPACT OF LYME DISEASE

The debilitating fatigue, arthritic pain, cognitive impairments, and other complications of chronic Lyme disease can come and go for many years, sometimes for a lifetime. These discussions examine some of the consequences of delayed treatment and undertreatment, including the soaring financial costs and preventable pain and suffering many patients bear.

COMPLICATIONS OF TICKBORNE DISEASES

Lyme disease and other tick-borne illnesses might make themselves known with the appearance of a circular rash with a spot in the center and a bout of flu-like illness. The patient may recall being bitten by a tick in the recent past. If he or she sees a doctor promptly, antibiotics are prescribed and the infection has the best chance of clearing. But many patients don't connect those early symptoms, or may not have them, and the disease appears to resolve on its own. Too often, in a month, a year, or several years, it reappears with far more serious complications. These include severe arthritis, fatigue, heart disease, neuropathy, depression, and cognitive deficiencies that mimic dementia. Lyme complications often then become chronic, particularly if they're undertreated or treated too late. The discussions look at common and less common complications. The case studies give a clearer picture of how these insidious impairments affect people's lives.

BABESIA PATIENTS CAN REMAIN SYMPTOMATIC FOR YEARS

*B*abesia can lead to serious illness. Patients have presented with atrial fibrillation,[116] noncardiogenic pulmonary edema,[117] and anemia.[116] In New York, between 1982 and 1991, seven people with Babesia died, while another patient on Nantucket Island developed pancarditis and died.[118]

Babesia can occur in the absence of old age, prior splenectomy (removal of the spleen), prematurity, immunosuppression, or liver disease.[116] Only five of 192 Babesia patients in one study were immunosuppressed.[119] None of the four Babesia subjects in another study had undergone a splenectomy.[116]

Babesia patients can remain symptomatic for years with constitutional, musculoskeletal, or neurological symptoms. One study found that 50 percent of coinfected patients were symptomatic for three months or longer, compared with only 4 percent of patients who had Lyme disease alone.[120] Meanwhile, one-third of patients with a history of both Babesia and Lyme disease remained symptomatic an average of six years.[116]

"The clinical pictures for 3 out of our 4 coinfected patients included a large number of symptoms, and 1 coinfected patient had persistent fatigue after treatment," according to a 2003 study by Steere and colleagues.[121]

Even when treated for Babesia, patients can die. New Jersey's former First Lady Jean Byrne (1974 to 1982), wife of former NJ governor Brendan Byrne, died in 2015, at the age of 88. Her obituary noted she "died from complications from Babesiosis, a tick-borne disease of the red blood cells after a brief illness."[122]

50

THE RISKS OF PAIN AND FATIGUE AFTER THREE WEEKS OF TREATMENT

Researchers at Johns Hopkins describe the risks of pain and fatigue after three weeks of doxycycline for an erythema migrans rash in the 2017 *Archives of Clinical Neuropsychology*[123]. Of 107 patients, 23 (21 percent) had a high fatigue total score and 33 of 107 patients (31 percent) had a high pain score. Five of 107 patients (5 percent) had a high depression total score.

The cutoffs for fatigue and pain were chosen to reflect clinically significant levels of each symptom based on the literature. A cutoff of 36 or greater was chosen for the Fatigue Severity Score (FSS) to indicate "high fatigue symptoms." A score of greater than 3 was chosen for the McGill Pain Scale to indicate "high pain symptoms." A total score of 13 or greater was chosen for the Beck Depression Inventory as indicating clinically significant symptoms of depression.

A substantial number of patients had a high level of symptoms immediately after completion of three weeks of doxycycline. "By the end of standard antibiotic treatment (Visit 2), those with high (clinically significant) symptoms of fatigue, pain, or depression continue to have impact on life functioning up to six months later," according to Bechtold and colleagues from the Department of

Physical Medicine and Rehabilitation, Johns Hopkins University School of Medicine, Baltimore, Md.

The researchers identified six individuals who suffered from post treatment Lyme disease syndrome (PTLDS). They used the Infectious Diseases Society of America (IDSA) case definition of PTLDS as follows:

"A documented episode of early or late Lyme disease with post-treatment resolution of objective signs of Lyme disease, but continuation or subsequent onset of symptoms of fatigue, widespread musculoskeletal pain, and/or complaints of cognitive difficulties. These subjective symptoms must be continuous or relapsing for at least six months following completion of treatment and must be severe enough to reduce the patient's functional ability."[123]

The remaining patients with severe fatigue and pain did not meet the IDSA criteria. It appears that studies of PTLDS following the IDSA criteria clearly underestimate the morbidity associated with Lyme disease.

The high number of patient suffering at six months after a three-week course of antibiotics for Lyme disease demonstrates the frustration of watchful waiting. Patients may be needlessly suffering for six months with pain, fatigue, and PTLDS. Patients may also find that treatment is more difficult after waiting for six months.

QUALITY OF LIFE FOR LYME DISEASE PATIENTS CAN BE GRIM

A clinical trial in the Netherlands titled "Persistent Lyme Empiric Antibiotic Study Europe (PLEASE)" found the quality of life for Lyme disease patients could be characterized as grim. Their quality of life was as poor as those found in four trials in the United States sponsored by the National Institutes of Health (NIH), using the SF-36 physical component of health (PCS) scale.[17,73,124]

The PCS measure of quality of life for Lyme patients was 31 to 32, worse than those of diabetic and cancer patients.[125] PCS scores for the general population are at least 50.[126]

Their PCS measure of quality of life rose by only 3 points, to less than 35, during the PLEASE trial, whether they were prescribed a two-week or 14-week course of antibiotics.[125]

The poor quality of life could be the result of enrolling patients who had been ill for a median of two years despite a median of two previous treatments.

Several options were not discussed. The study investigators could have enrolled patients who had not been sick for years or failed previous treatments. They could also have called for better outcomes.[125,127,128] And they could have encouraged doctors to avoid treatment delays, which averaged 1.9 years.[125]

The PLEASE investigators could have prescribed four weeks of IV ceftriaxone instead of two weeks[16,68], given that four weeks of IV ceftriaxone has already been shown to be more effective for chronic manifestations of Lyme disease.

Four weeks of IV ceftriaxone was more effective than placebo in one of the Krupp NIH-sponsored clinical trials.[73] Ten weeks of IV ceftriaxone was more effective than placebo for fatigue but not for cognitive function in the Fallon NIH-sponsored clinical trial.[17]

The PLEASE investigators also could have developed individualized treatment regimens based on each patient's clinical response. Finally, the investigators could have recommended evaluations for co-infections (e.g., *Babesia*).[58]

FATIGUE CAN BE SEVERE IN LYME DISEASE

Fatigue can be severe in acute and chronic presentations of Lyme disease. Fatigue may be a component of an acute sickness reaction with elevated proinflammatory cytokines."[129]

Fatigue has also been described in chronic manifestations of Lyme disease. It was one of the most common symptoms in chronic neurologic Lyme disease,[16] Lyme encephalopathy,[17,68] post Lyme disease,[73] and post-treatment Lyme disease syndrome.[130,131]

Severe fatigue was successfully treated in two randomized clinical trial of patients with persistent illness after treatment. In a study by Krupp and colleagues of post-treatment Lyme disease, improvements at six months on the Fatigue Severity Scale (FSS-11) was noted for 64 percent of patients who received one month of IV ceftriaxone.[73]

In Fallon and colleague's randomized clinical trials of patients with Lyme encephalopathy, on post hoc comparison, improvement at six months on the FSS-11 scale was noted for 66.7 percent of patients who received 10 weeks of IV ceftriaxone vs. 25 percent who received IV placebo (Fisher exact test, $p = 0.05$).[17]

DOES LYME DISEASE AFFECT YOUR ABILITY TO WORK?

In a study of 27 patients with chronic neurologic Lyme disease, most were able to remain employed. Three of them quit their jobs, three decreased their workload to part time, and two retired early, according to Logigian and colleagues from the Tufts University School of Medicine. They reported their findings in *The New England Journal of Medicine* in 1990[16]

Another study, published in *Emerging Infectious Diseases*, described the costs for chronic Lyme disease patients living in five counties along the eastern shore of Maryland between 1997 and 2000.[132] Investigators found that more than 50 percent of their costs were caused by loss of productivity. Total costs for chronic Lyme disease patients was $16,199 annually; $8,785 of that was attributed to losses in productivity.[132]

"We used patient-reported time lost from work to estimate productivity losses due to Lyme disease on the basis of the human capital method and valued the time lost by using age- and sex-weighted productivity valuation tables," says Zhang from the Centers for Disease Control and Prevention.[132]

For patients younger than 15, researchers assumed that their parents (usually the mothers) had to take time off from work to take care of them. The values of their mothers' lost days of work were included.

The risk of Lyme disease impacting work and its potential risk to the workforce bolsters the need to introduce more effective treatment options.

54

BOTH MEN AND WOMAN CAN SUFFER FOR YEARS AFTER TREATMENT

*E*leven percent of individuals diagnosed with Lyme disease, followed for a decade, suffered at least once with post-treatment Lyme disease syndrome.[131]

The study by Weitzner and colleagues concludes that males and females with "culture-confirmed early Lyme disease had similar clinical features, rates of seropositivity, and long-term outcomes."[131] Women (12.3 percent) and men (9.9 percent) both suffered from post-treatment Lyme disease syndrome.[131]

Post-treatment Lyme disease syndrome occurred despite prompt treatment. In the Weitzner study, the women were ill an average of 5.28 days before treatment began, while men were sick 7.09 days.[131]

The study may have underestimated the risk of post-treatment Lyme disease syndrome because 60 percent of the patients were lost to follow-up.

There is no evidence whether patients with post-treatment Lyme disease syndrome were retreated with antibiotics for their original infection.

55

SOME LYME DISEASE PATIENTS DO WELL

A 2016 longitudinal study gives the appearance that there are no complications of Lyme disease. "Both mental health and physical health scores increased to be at or above national average over time, regardless of Lyme disease stage or severity at diagnosis,"[133] according to Wills and colleagues from the National Institute of Allergy and Infectious Diseases, National Institutes of Health, writing in the journal *Clinical Infectious Diseases*.

The outcomes from the study were far better than expected because patients with pre-existing comorbidities and symptoms similar to post-treatment Lyme disease syndrome were excluded from the study.[134] Samples are biased if they omit any group of people from participating in research protocols.

At the very least, the study showed some Lyme patients do well after treatment for Lyme disease. The question the study didn't answer was why.

56

MORE THAN HALF OF PATIENTS WITH LYME NEUROBORRELIOSIS ILL FOR YEARS

Dersch and colleagues reported that more than 17 of 30 subjects (57 percent)[135] with "definite" Lyme neuroborreliosis reported residual symptoms an average of 5.7 years after antibiotic treatment. The residual symptoms consisted of pain (n = 6), ataxia (n = 6), sensory disturbances (n = 4), cranial nerve disorder (n = 2), spastic gait (n = 2), fatigue (n = 2), and micturition disorder (n = 1).[135]

Their 30 patients had compatible neurological symptoms, CSF pleocytosis, antibodies against *Borrelia burgdorferi* in serum and CSF, and a CSF/serum antibody index of at least 2.[135] The 30 patients had initially been treated at the Medical Center, University of Freiburg, between 2003 and 2014[135] an average of 4.1 weeks after onset of symptoms with either ceftriaxone, doxycycline, or both antibiotics.[135]

Their 17 "definite" Lyme neuroborreliosis patients with residual symptoms presented with an average Fatigue Severity Scale (FSS) score of 4.29.[73] Krupp and colleagues defined severe fatigue as 4.0 or higher in a clinical trial sponsored by the National Institutes of Health.[73]

Their 17 "definite" Lyme neuroborreliosis patients with residual symptoms also presented with poor quality of life. "Patients with residual symptoms had statistically significantly lower measures of quality of life, as measured with the physical component summary of the SF-36 compared to patients without residual symptoms," according to Dersch and colleagues.[135] "The proportion of patients with residual symptoms is similar to proportions reported in other studies of antibiotically treated" patients with Lyme neuroborreliosis, say Dersch and others.[135] The 17 patients did not present with depression or global cognitive impairment.

For some reason, Dersch and colleagues overlooked the severe fatigue and poor quality of life for their "definite" Lyme neuroborreliosis patients who remained ill when coming to the following conclusion. "Our results do not support the hypothesis that a considerable proportion of patients with antibiotically treated [Lyme neuroborreliosis] develops a 'post Lyme syndrome' consisting of debilitating fatigue or cognitive impairment or have severe limitations of quality of life."[135]

Dersch and colleagues may have overlooked the severe fatigue and poor quality of life by pooling the results of the 17 patients with "definite" Lyme neuroborreliosis with the 13 patients without persistent symptoms.[135]

The cause of the poor outcomes for their "definite" Lyme neuroborreliosis subjects was not addressed. Furthermore, the study was not designed to assess whether more than four weeks of initial therapy might have improved outcomes.

THE TREATMENT COSTS OF LYME DISEASE CAN BE SIGNIFICANT FOR PATIENTS

The costs of Lyme disease can be significant for patients. A study identified Lyme disease cases based on the physicians' determination in the medical record, clinical findings, tick exposure, and other relevant details (e.g., laboratory test results). The cases were collected between 1997 and 2000 from patients living in five counties along the eastern shore of Maryland, an area endemic for Lyme disease.[132]

The mean costs for early Lyme disease were $1,310 consisting of $801 for direct medical costs, $259 for indirect medical costs, $52 for nonmedical costs, and $198 for lost productivity costs.[132]

The costs of Lyme disease were much higher for individuals with chronic manifestations. The mean cost for those patients was $16,199 annually. Costs consisted of $1,872 for direct medical costs, $434 for indirect medical costs, $5,109 for nonmedical costs, and $8,785 for lost productivity.[132]

The annual cost per-patient with chronic manifestations of Lyme disease was higher than the cost for other common chronic illnesses:

$10,716 for rheumatoid arthritis,[136] $10,911 for fibromyalgia,[136] and $13,094 for lupus.[137]

LYME DISEASE COULD COST SOCIETY BILLIONS

Estimating the total cost of Lyme disease to society is no small challenge, given controversies over the number of cases and the disease's long-term consequences. Zhang and colleagues, at the Centers for Disease Control and Prevention (CDC), set out to estimate the financial impact of only those cases reported to the CDC in a single year. The year was 2002, when 23,763 cases of Lyme disease were reported to the CDC.

Zhang and colleagues estimated that the national economic impact of Lyme disease and relevant complaints was about $203 million (all costs in 2002 dollars).[132]

The authors postulated that the financial impact of Lyme disease would be significantly higher if the actual number of cases were considered. The CDC estimated that the actual number of new cases of Lyme disease to be at least 300,000 a year in 2013.[138]

If just one-third of those 2013 cases developed chronic manifestations, the total annual cost of Lyme disease would be as much as $2 billion.

Here's the math; assuming about one third of the 300,000, or 100,000

Lyme disease patients, developed chronic manifestations each year, as estimated by Asch, Shadick, and Aucott. .[76,77,130]

Of those 300,000 patients, 192,000 would develop early Lyme disease for a one-time cost of about $1,310, or $251 million total.

The remaining 108,000 patients (the approximate 1/3) would develop chronic Lyme disease at an annual cost of $16,199, or $1.75 billion total for the first year alone.

That brings the total cost to society for all 300,000 patients to about $2 billion.

Two important considerations: First, Zhang and colleagues' numbers do not reflect future costs beyond the one-year study period. That means the $2 billion cost calculated here (in 2002 dollars) reflects only one year's costs to society. About 11 percent of the patients would suffer from post-treatment Lyme disease syndrome at least once during the decade after treatment for culture-confirmed early Lyme disease.[131] Thus, the cost to individuals who remain ill for decades is unknown.

Second, pain and suffering were not accounted for in the study.

So, how much does Lyme disease really cost? The answer is quite a lot of money for both individuals and society. Such high costs support the urgent need for more effective treatment regimens than a one-time, two- to three-week course of antibiotics. Watchful waiting is a risky and costly strategy in dealing with the Lyme disease epidemic.

A SECOND STUDY PUTS COSTS AT UP TO $1.3 BILLION A YEAR

Another study, this one from 2015, found our healthcare system is spending between $712 million and $1.3 billion each year to treat Lyme disease and lingering illnesses associated with it. Researchers from the Johns Hopkins Bloomberg School of Public Health[139] published "Healthcare Costs, Utilization and Patterns of Care Following Lyme Disease" in *PLOS ONE*.[139] They also suggest that Lyme disease is more debilitating and widespread than previously thought.[139]

They estimated that 240,000 to 440,000 people are diagnosed with Lyme disease each year, with an average of $3,000 spent annually per patient on treatment. "Our study looks at the actual costs of treating patients in the year following their Lyme diagnosis," say Adrion and colleagues. This includes repeated medical visits and diagnostic tests for symptoms that have not resolved after the initial course of antibiotic treatment.

"It is clear that we need effective, cost-effective and compassionate management of these patients to improve their outcomes even if we don't know what to call the disease," according to the authors.[140] "Regardless of what you call it, our data show that many people who have been diagnosed with Lyme disease are, in fact, going back to the doctor complaining of persistent symptoms, getting multiple tests and being re-treated."[139]

The severity of chronic symptoms after Lyme disease treatment and the size of the patient population affected may be vastly underestimated. In fact, the study found 63 percent of those treated for Lyme disease reported at least one subsequent related diagnosis, a rate 36 percentage points higher than those who did not have Lyme disease. The CDC reports that only 10 percent to 20 percent of patients experience lingering symptoms after completing 2- to 4-week antibiotic regimes for Lyme disease.[139]

The Johns Hopkins researchers also report that individuals with Lyme disease were 5.5 times more likely to have a diagnosis of debility and excessive fatigue. And within the year following the Lyme disease diagnosis, patients had 87 percent more visits to the doctor and 71 percent more visits to the emergency room than matched controls.[139]

SECTION VI. LIMITATIONS OF LABORATORY TESTS

Accurate, timely tests for Lyme disease, and especially for the more recently discovered related diseases like Babesia, are sorely lacking. Even the ticks themselves can be poor predictors of the infections they spread. The result: Lyme disease and its tick-borne cousins are often misdiagnosed for other illnesses. And some physicians don't even test for Lyme when symptoms should raise strong suspicions of the disease. The discussions that follow look at the vexing performance of available tests and at some of the conditions mistakenly diagnosed when Lyme disease is the true culprit.

82 PERCENT OF STUDY PATIENTS WITH CLINICAL HISTORY OF LYME NOT TESTED

A study out of Duke University Health System in Durham, North Carolina revealed that only 18% of the patients who had sought treatment for Lyme disease at Duke, and had a "clinical history consistent with Lyme disease", had actually been tested for the infection.[141] According to Lantos et.al., only 297 patients of the 1,621 individuals who sought treatment for Lyme through the health care system between 2005 and 2010 were actually sent for lab tests. The study results were published in the July 2015 issue of *Clinical Infectious Diseases*.[141]

The 297 tested patients were described as follows:[141]

- 110 patients with arthritis of a large joint
- 98 patients with cranial nerve palsy
- 75 patients with meningitis
- 11 patients with both meningitis and cranial neuropathy
- one patient with both arthritis and cranial nerve palsy
- one patient with atrioventricular block
- one patient with both atrioventricular block and cranial nerve palsy

The study does not explain why 82 percent of individuals with clinical histories "consistent with Lyme disease" were not tested.

Moreover, the study does not indicate whether it included individuals with other manifestations of Lyme disease, such as chronic neurologic Lyme disease,[16] Lyme encephalopathy,[17,68] neuropsychiatric Lyme disease,[18] and post-treatment Lyme disease.[19]

This study should serve as a reminder of the need for clinicians to evaluate any patient with a clinical history consistent with Lyme disease in North Carolina and elsewhere to determine if they have the illness.

DOCTORS ARE NOT TESTING FOR BABESIA AND ANAPLASMOSIS

In an effort to begin to understand what kinds of tests doctors were ordering in an attempt to diagnose tick-borne infections in patients, researchers examined data from seven large commercial laboratories, as well as data "from another 1051 smaller commercial, hospital, and government laboratories in four states (CT, MD, MN, and NY)." The researchers wanted to know what tests doctors had ordered other than Lyme tests. The data examined was collected in 2008, and at the time, these four states had some of the highest incidents of tick infections in the country.[142]

The seven commercial labs tested 2,927,881 specimens from around the United States.[142] Among those more than 2.9M specimens, only "495,585 specimens or (17%) were tested for tick-borne diseases other than Lyme disease." Among the smaller labs contacted, 92 of the total 1051 reported back providing data which showed these labs had tested "a total of 10,091 specimens for four tick-borne diseases other than Lyme disease."

A further examination of all the collected data revealed six percent, or 193,121 tests, were ordered for Ehrlichiosis. Three percent, or 85,323 tests, were ordered for Babesia. Less than 3 percent, or 63,693 tests, were ordered for Anaplasmosis. Less than one percent, or 3,750 specimens, were ordered for the combination of Ehrlichiosis and Anaplasmosis. No tests were ordered for Powassan encephalitis.

The seven participating labs were ARUP, Clinical Laboratory Partners, Focus Diagnostics, Laboratory Corporation of America (LabCorp), Mayo Clinic Laboratories, Quest Diagnostics, and Specialty Laboratories. "None of the laboratories known to perform alternative testing agreed to participate," according to Hinckley and colleagues from the Division of Vector-Borne Diseases, Centers for Disease Control and Prevention, Fort Collins, Colo.[142]

While nearly three million specimens were examined, readers are probably wondering why doctors in these four endemic states (CT, MD, MN, and NY) didn't order more tests for co-infections. Had the laboratories known to perform alternative testing had participated, researchers might have actually found more testing was done for other tick-borne infections.

The authors even noted some surprise that nationally, more tests were ordered for "ehrlichiosis than for RMSF" and this increased testing for Ehrlichiosis came about, "despite the fact that more than twice the number of RMSF cases were reported to CDC in 2008 than ehrlichiosis cases."

The authors noted the 2008 data from this study served as "a baseline to evaluate trends in tick-borne disease test utilization and insight into the burden of these diseases."

Going forward, it would be interesting to see how testing for co-infections has changed over time, especially since Babesia became a nationally notifiable illness in 2011. At the very least, the research shows the importance of testing patients for co-infections of Lyme disease.

TESTING ENGORGED TICKS NOT RELIABLE

One would assume that engorged ticks would be more likely to be positive for *Borrelia burgdorferi* infections than unengorged ticks. Instead, the engorged ticks had a lower rate of *B. burgdorferi* infections, according to a study by Gasmi and colleagues from the Institut National de Santé Publique du Québec.

In that study, 24.9 percent of unengorged ticks were positive, compared with only 8.9 percent of engorged ticks.[143] Researchers tested 4,596 *Ixodes scapularis* ticks removed from humans in Quebec between 2008 and 2014. The study was published in the *Journal of Ticks and Tick-borne Diseases*.

The findings are consistent with those from another Canadian study that also collected ticks from humans.[144]

The lower rate of *B. burgdorferi* in engorged ticks could result from an inhibitor in the blood meal.[145] "Perhaps this was due to simpler reasons such as the greater likelihood that unengorged ticks remained alive up to DNA extraction, while engorged ticks may well have died days or weeks before testing," note the authors.[143]

In any case, testing engorged ticks may not be a reliable tool in determining a patient's risk of infection. This is disappointing, given that engorged ticks are more likely to transmit Lyme disease.

BLOOD SMEARS UNRELIABLE FOR DIAGNOSING BABESIA

Clinicians cannot rely on blood smears in making a diagnosis of babesiosis. "Parasites frequently cannot be seen in blood film,"[60] explain Krause and colleagues from the Departments of Pediatrics and Laboratory Medicine, University of Connecticut School of Medicine, Farmington, Conn. In their New England study, the serologic tests for Babesia pathogens were negative in 67 percent of patients by microscopic evaluation, in 29 percent of patients by specific amplifiable DNA, and in 22 percent of patients by antibodies.[119]

"Physicians caring for patients with moderate to severe Lyme disease should consider obtaining diagnostic tests for Babesia and possibly other tick-borne pathogens in regions where these diseases are zoonotic, especially in patients experiencing episodes of 'atypical Lyme disease' or patients in whom the response to antibiotic treatment is delayed or absent," urge Krause and colleagues.

Identifying Babesia is critical since treatment is different than that for Lyme disease. "For the treatment of babesiosis, a regimen of atovaquone and azithromycin is as effective as a regimen of clindamycin and quinine and is associated with fewer adverse reactions," write Krause and colleagues.[146]

CHRONIC INFLAMMATORY DEMYELINATING POLYNEUROPATHY CASE SEROCONVERTS TO LYME DISEASE

*L*yme disease can often be ruled out as a comorbid condition based on negative serologic tests, only to seroconvert to positive on follow-up. [147,148] That's exactly what happened in the case of a woman diagnosed with chronic inflammatory demyelinating polyneuropathy (CIDP). Lyme disease was ruled out based on negative serologic testing but seroconverted to positive on follow-up testing, according to Perronne and colleagues from the Versailles Saint Quentin University, Garches, France.

The patient, a 41-year-old woman presented with asthenia (lack of energy), weakness, and diffuse paresthesia (tingling or numbness). The electromyography assessment showed mild demyelination. Lyme disease was rule out based on negative serum and cerebrospinal fluid serologic tests.

Intravenous immunoglobulin treatment was performed eight times for CIDP, with subsequent partial response and relapse.

Lyme disease was diagnosed 10 months after the onset of clinical symptoms, when a serum polymerase chain reaction analysis disclosed the presence of *Borrelia* (100 copies/mL).

Lyme disease was successfully treated with six weeks of a combination of doxycycline and hydroxychloroquine. The 41-year-old patient showed "a dramatic clinical improvement," along with "complete disappearance of the neurologic signs," according to Perronne and colleagues.

The authors advise against automatically ruling out Lyme disease based on negative serologic tests. "In our opinion," noted the authors, "Lyme formal serology negativity is insufficient to rule out early (erythema migrans) and late chronic Lyme disease diagnosis." [147]

LYME DISEASE CAUSES A POSITIVE TEST FOR MONO

When does a patient have mononucleosis and when does a patient have Lyme disease? And can one disease look like the other? Those are the questions raised in a paper by Pavlectic and colleagues. "We report two cases of false positive Epstein-Barr virus (EBV) serologies in early-disseminated Lyme disease," wrote the National Institute of Mental Health researchers in the journal *Clinical Infectious Diseases*. [149]

In the first case, a 16-year-old male from Virginia developed fatigue, myalgias, and three brief episodes of fevers over an 18-day period. Acute infectious mononucleosis was diagnosed based on a positive viral capsid antigen (VCA) IgM and negative VCA IgG. [149]

Lyme disease was diagnosed 17 days later with multiple erythematous rashes and right-sided peripheral facial nerve palsy. Laboratory evaluation revealed a positive C6 peptide, ELISA index of 6.02, and a positive IgM immunoblot. A four-week course of doxycycline was successful. [149]

"Repeat VCA IgG, VCA IgM, and Epstein-Barr nuclear antigen

(EBNA) were negative, indicating that the initial VCA IgM was falsely positive," the researchers noted. [149]

In the second case, an avid biker from Maryland presented with a six-day history of fatigue, fever, myalgia, and headache. Lyme disease was diagnosed the next day based on multiple erythematous rashes. Lyme serologies were positive by ELISA, IgG, and IgM immunoblots.

Twelve days into the patient's illness, she tested positive for mononucleosis with a positive VCA IgM, VCA IgG, EBV early antigen, EBNA IgG, and positive monospot.

The fever resolved and the rashes faded with a 21-day course of doxycycline. The recovery was complicated by a right upper trunk brachial plexopathy. "The pain resolved and the weakness improved over the next six months," according to the authors. [149]

"Three and a half years later, repeat VCA IgG and EBNA were positive, and VCA IgM was negative," according to Pavletic and colleagues. [149]

Both cases were initially misdiagnosed, according to the authors. "Here we present two cases where early manifestations of Lyme disease were initially misdiagnosed as acute EBV infection due to positive VCA IgM results," they say. [149]

The authors touch on the difficulty of interpreting acute mononucleosis testing. "While isolated VCA IgM may indicate early acute mononucleosis, the test can be nonspecific, especially when the likelihood of acute EBV infection is low," according to Pavletic and colleagues. They add, "Immune activation with other pathogens can also result in a false positive VCA IgM. [149]

The second case was difficult to interpret given the positive monospot, heterophile, and VCA IgM tests. "In this case, we cannot exclude that the positive VCA IgM could be due to subclinical EBV reactivation, which has little clinical relevance in immunocompetent individuals," according to Pavletic and colleagues. They add,

"Heterophile antibody tests are known to have false positives due to acute infections, autoimmune diseases, and cancer." [149]

In practice, Lyme disease and mono are common conditions that share similar symptoms. The authors' two cases remind us of the need to consider Lyme disease even if initial serologies suggest mono.

DON'T ELIMINATE LAB-DEVELOPED TEST FOR TICKBORNE ILLNESSES

*T*he tick populations are expanding to new regions, and complex vector-borne organisms are emerging, posing threats to public health. The U.S. Food and Drug Administration's attempt to eliminate lab-developed tests for tick-borne diseases could stifle innovation and discourage researchers and pathologists from searching for solutions. In the end, the growing number of patients with Lyme disease will pay the price, as will all those still undiagnosed.

For example, *Borrelia miyamotoi* is a relatively new bacterium that can cause relapsing fever and symptoms like those of Lyme disease. The bacterium was only recently identified, in 2011, in Russia and has since been found in the Netherlands, Japan, and the northeastern United States and California. [150-152]

Researchers have had to diagnose *B. miyamotoi* based on blood smear,[153] direct detection of spirochetes using polymerase chain reaction (PCR),[154,155] or a recombinant glycerophosphodiester phosphodiesterase (rGlpQ) protein.[65]

Lab-developed tests for *B. miyamotoi* have not been approved by the

FDA. And if the FDA gets its way, physicians would have access only to diagnostic tests for tick-borne diseases that it has approved. This could limit the clinician's ability to diagnose Lyme disease and other tick-borne co-infections — a risky move when we're seeing an emergence of multiple tick-borne pathogens.

SERONEGATIVE B. MIYAMOTOI

"Infection with *Borrelia miyamotoi* is the fifth recognized *Ixodes*-transmitted infection in the northeastern United States and should be part of the differential diagnosis of febrile patients from areas where deer-tick-transmitted infections are endemic,"[65] according to Molloy and colleagues from IMUGEN, a Norwood, Massachusetts based lab.[65]

Researchers initially identified cases of *B. miyamotoi* by whole-blood polymerase chain reaction (PCR) for common tick-borne infections in Massachusetts, New Jersey, New York, and Rhode Island. [65]

Most of the patients presented with headaches, myalgias, arthralgias, and malaise/fatigue. "More than 50 percent were suspected of having sepsis, and 24 percent required hospitalization," according to Molloy and colleagues.[65]

The poor sensitivity of the whole-blood PCR or rGlpQ for *B. miyamotoi* in the study arguably could be called seronegative *B. miyamotoi*. The recombinant glycerophosphodiester phosphodiesterase (rGlpQ) protein test was negative for most of the cases of *B. miyamotoi* when initially treated. "Serologic testing using the rGlpQ EIA seems insensitive in diagnosing acute *B. miyamotoi* infection given that it was positive for IgG or IgM in only 16 percent of the case patient samples at the time of clinical presentation," say the authors.[65]

The rGlpQ was positive after the fact in 86 percent of the patients during convalescence.[65]

B. miyamotoi disease may be clinically similar to or be confused with human anaplasmosis, according to Molloy and colleagues.[65] He adds that elevated liver enzyme levels, neutropenia, and thrombocytopenia were seen 75 percent, 60 percent, and 51 percent of the time, respectively.

SECTION VII. CHALLENGES OF DIAGNOSING THE DISEASE

Prompt diagnosis of Lyme and related diseases matters. The longer patients go without diagnosis and treatment, the more likely their disease will get worse and persist longer. Given the limits and unreliability of available tests, it's expected that diagnosing Lyme disease and related tick-borne illnesses is a difficult task. Diagnosis is further complicated by co-infections, with symptoms that mimic other common diseases. As the discussions show here, practicing physicians often must rely on their clinical judgement, and good communication with their patients, to diagnose this exasperating disease.

LYME DISEASE INITIALLY DIAGNOSED AS JUVENILE RHEUMATOID ARTHRITIS

Lyme disease was first identified in 1975 in a group of children and adolescents living in Lyme, Connecticut who suffered from recurrent attacks of asymmetric swelling and pain in the knee. The patients were initially diagnosed with juvenile rheumatoid arthritis.

"The typical patient has had three recurrences, but 16 patients have had none," noted lead investigator Steere, then a postdoctoral fellow in rheumatology at Yale University.[5] "During remission, some patients remembered short periods of joint pain, sometimes lasting only hours, without swelling (and therefore, not included as attacks)."

Pain also occurred in the ankle, wrist, temporomandibular joint, shoulder, hip, and elbow. Other symptoms included malaise, fatigue, headaches, myalgia, periorbital edema, and swelling of the hands or feet. Of the 12 subjects, seven suffered from "profound fatigue and hyperesthesia, sometimes persisting for months after the arthritis had gone," say Steere and colleagues.[5]

A team of researchers including Steere would, 14 years later, report in the *New England Journal of Medicine* that chronic neurologic Lyme disease was one of the complications of Lyme disease.[16]

CASE STUDY: AMERICAN WOMAN DIAGNOSED AFTER TRAVELING TO COLUMBIA

Travelers typically prepare to possibly incur infections when visiting other countries. A case study in *Travel Medicine Infectious Diseases* titled "American Woman with Early Lyme Borreliosis Diagnosed in a Colombian Hospital" reminds travelers that they should not overlook an infection they may have contracted from their country of origin.[156]

Doctors in Bogotá, Colombia describe an encounter with a 24-year-old American woman whom they eventually diagnosed with Lyme disease seven days after she arrived in the country from Virginia.[156]

The woman presented to a Bogotá emergency room with a "popular pruritic lesion in [the] right flank." The patient told the emergency room physician that a week earlier, she had walked through the woods with her dog and had noticed a dark spot in the center of where a rash appeared.

She was initially prescribed oral cephalexin for a presumed cellulitis.[156] Cephalexin is not effective for the treatment of Lyme disease.[90]

The next day, the hospital's infectious disease department diagnosed

Lyme disease based on her 27-cm target-like rash, malaise, headache, arthralgia and abdominal pain, exposure history, and origin. Doxycycline was prescribed (100 mg every 12 hours) for 10 days. The rash and symptoms resolved by day 7.[156]

The American woman was fortunate enough to present with a classic target-like erythema migrans rash. The challenge for doctors in Bogata was to diagnose Lyme disease brought into their country from America. American doctors face similar challenges when treating visiting travelers from abroad. What disease was acquired during the visit? What disease was pre-existing when arriving in the country?

70

DON'T COUNT ON A RELAPSING FEVER TO DIAGNOSE B. MIYAMOTOI

You might assume a patient infected with *Borrelia miyamotoi*, a relapsing fever spirochete, to present with a relapsing fever. However, your assumption would be wrong 48 out of 50 times, according to a case series published in the *Annals of Internal Medicine*.[65] The authors found that only two out of 50 patients infected with the relapsing spirochete *B. miyamotoi* actually presented with a relapsing fever.[65]

B. miyamotoi has the genetic apparatus for antigenic variation (meaning the pathogen can adapt to avoid detection by the immune system) that typically drives relapsing fevers, according to Sudhindra and colleagues from the Division of Infectious Diseases, New York Medical College.[157] Nevertheless, relapsing fevers have not been demonstrated clinically or in an animal system for *B. miyamotoi*."

All but one of the 51 individuals in the case series presented with a fever. The study authors wrote, "The low percentage of cases with a relapse of fever may be due to the frequent use of empiric antibiotic therapy early in the course of febrile illnesses in patients with tick exposures."[157]

CASE STUDY: FIRST REPORT OF MALARIA WITH LYME DISEASE AS A COINFECTION

Malaria and Lyme disease are common vector-borne illnesses. Malaria is considered a tropical parasite and Lyme disease is a non-tropical bacterium. Yet, doctors in Portugal documented both conditions in a 41-year-old patient, according to a study published in the 2017 *Clinical Case Reports*.[158]

"As far as we are aware, we are writing the first report of *Plasmodium* spp. and *Borrelia burgdorferi* co-infection (a co-infection of a tropical parasite and a nontropical bacterium)," according to Neves and colleagues from the Infectious Diseases Department, Centro Hospitalar São João, Porto, Portugal.[158]

Malaria was suspected based on the man having returned to Portugal from Angola, where he worked as a welder. Malaria was diagnosed based on examination of thin blood films and a rapid diagnostic testing for malaria. The diagnosis of mixed-*Plasmodium* was made based on subsequent finding of *Plasmodium spp.*[158]

The Portuguese doctors discovered Lyme disease during their evaluation for neurological symptoms. "The concomitant diagnosis of borreliosis was based on clinical presentation and positive serology for *B. burgdorferi* sensu lato," according to the authors. "Positive PCR for *B. burgdorferi* sensu lato in CSF [cerebral spinal fluid] also confirmed neuroborreliosis," they add.

The treatment changed after recognizing the co-infection with Lyme disease. The initial antimalarial treatment consisted of intravenous quinine, 600 mg every eight hours, and IV doxycycline, 100 mg every 12 hours. Intravenous ceftriaxone, 2 g every 12 hours was added to the therapeutic regimen for 14 days after recognition of the Lyme disease. The patient also required treatment for an autolimited antiphospholipid syndrome.[158]

Neves and colleagues point out the importance of considering co-infections. "Atypical malaria has a broad differential diagnosis, of which co-infections represent a cornerstone. Making such a diagnosis is of vital importance in terms of management and prognosis. This is particularly true in the case of the co-infection of *B. burgdorferi*, due to the potentially devastating neurological and systemic manifestations and the therapeutic implications."[158]

WHY WAS THE LEVEL OF HOSPITAL DIAGNOSES HIGH DURING THE WINTER IN ENGLAND?

A 2017 study reported a 42 percent increase in the number of Lyme disease hospital diagnoses in England from 2011 to 2015. Cooper and colleagues report those results in the *British Journal of General Practice* based on hospital episode statistics data in England from the Health and Social Care Information Centre.[159] Some patients may have been admitted more than once.

While the study reports a high level of hospital-based diagnoses year-round, the authors were unable to discern the reasons for an increase during the winter months. The data for the study was entered by non-clinical coders and therefore was inadequate.

The authors suggest that the high level of winter diagnoses might reflect the milder winters associated with climate change. The high level of diagnoses might also reflect hospital admissions other than an erythema migrans rash, such as neurologic manifestations.

The Lyme disease cases identified in England using hospital episode statistics should encourage further study. "A heightened awareness of risk may facilitate appropriate prophylaxis, diagnosis, and treatment," according to Cooper and colleagues.[159]

BABESIA DIFFICULT TO DIAGNOSE

Babesia can be difficult to diagnose with current serologic testing. The parasite was detected microscopically in as few as one-third of patients with Babesia.[119] Specific amplifiable DNA and IgM antibodies were more likely to be positive.[118] The reliability of serologic tests for Babesia in actual practice remains to be determined.

The Babesia tests can be false negative. There may be too few Babesia sporozoites to be detected on a thin smear, or the infection can resolve with or without treatment. It's been reported that a positive serologic test for *B. microti* will decay over time, leading to a negative test. Half of the patients with positive serologic tests for Babesia were negative on follow-up.[116]

SWEATS MAY BE HELPFUL IN DIAGNOSING BABESIA

Sweats have been reported in patients with babesiosis.[160] This finding should come as no surprise given that babesiosis is related to malaria, a vector-borne disease that also causes of sweats. Nearly half of the patients (46 percent) in a New England study who presented with a combination of Babesia and Lyme disease reported having sweats.[60]

Krause and colleagues report their findings in 1996 in the *Journal of the American Medical Association*.[60] The authors note that in addition to sweats, their patients suffered symptoms including fatigue (81 percent), headache (77 percent), fever (58 percent), chills (42 percent), myalgia (38 percent), anorexia (31 percent), arthralgia (27 percent), emotional lability (23 percent), and neck stiffness (23 percent).

While sweats may be helpful in diagnosing Babesia, physicians can't fully rely on the symptom. Sweats can also be absent. In the Krause study, 42 percent of babesiosis patients did not have sweats. Furthermore, sweats have been reported in other tick-borne illnesses. Studies by Krause and Ramsey found 22 percent of patients with Lyme disease and 37.5 percent of patients with anaplasmosis complained of sweats.[146,161]

When evaluating patients suspected of having Babesia, the physician's clinical judgment is still the best diagnostic tool.

Note that sweats have also been reported in a variety of other conditions. "Night-time sweating has been associated with menopause, malignancies, autoimmune diseases, and infections," according to Mold and colleagues from the College of Medicine, University of Oklahoma Health Sciences Center.[162]

SIGNS OF LYME DISEASE MAY DISAPPEAR THEN RE-EMERGE

*L*yme disease complications may not be apparent at the end of the initial course of treatment. The signs can disappear only to re-emerge at a different time. The recurrence of Lyme disease has been referred to as a relapse.

The duration of the latent period to a relapse can be variable and prolonged.[16,68,163] Strle from the University Medical Centre, Department of Infectious Diseases, Ljubljana, Slovenia reported a relapse at 20 months.[164] Logigian from the Department of Neurology, Tufts University School of Medicine described a median time from an erythema migrans rash to chronic neurologic Lyme disease of 26 months, with a range of 1–168 months.[16]

"Signs of Lyme disease disappeared post-treatment; however, new-onset patient-reported symptoms increased or plateaued over time," note Aucott and colleagues in 2013 in *Quality of Life Research*. "At 6 months, 36 percent of patients reported new-onset fatigue, 20 percent widespread pain, and 45 percent neurocognitive difficulties."[19]

UP TO 40 PERCENT OF LYME DISEASE PATIENTS ARE INFECTED WITH BABESIA

Although Lyme disease is the most talked about tick-transmitted disease, babesiosis is more common than you might think. In the 2015 issue of *Trends in Parasitology*, Diuk-Wasser and colleagues report that up to 40 percent of patients with Lyme disease experienced concurrent babesiosis.[58]

This means that out of the estimated 300,000 cases of Lyme disease reported annually in the United States, 120,000 of the patients may also have Babesia. This is particularly alarming given that the disease can go undetected in asymptomatic individuals and is transmissible congenitally or through blood transfusions.[165]

Babesia cannot be treated with the same medications used for Lyme disease, either. Doxycycline is effective for treating Lyme disease, Ehrlichiosis, and Anaplasmosis, but not for Babesia. Treatment with Mepron and Zithromax has been effective for Babesia. Quinine and clindamycin have also been effective but are associated with a higher rate of side effects. Flagyl and Tindamax have been described but not evaluated in trials. The optimal regimen for Babesia continues to be debated.

CASE STUDY: 70-YEAR-OLD MAN ILL WITH BABESIOSIS AND LYME DISEASE

A 70-year-old man with a four-day history of headaches, high fevers, nonbilious vomiting, and low urine output was described in a case report in the 2015 *Quarterly Journal of Medicine*.[166] Babesia was considered based on a six-month history of living with his daughter in eastern Long Island, N.Y. Malaria was also considered, given he had emigrated from Bangladesh six months prior to becoming ill.

Laboratory tests supported the Babesia diagnosis. "Peripheral blood smear revealed intracellular ovoid rings resembling both Plasmodium sp. and *B. microti* rings," state Zaiem and colleagues from the Mayo Evidence-Based Practice Center, Mayo Clinic. The PCR test came back positive for *B. microti* and the patient was started on a seven-day treatment with doxycycline and quinine to cover either infection. He showed improvement in both symptoms and laboratory findings.

Just prior to being discharged from the hospital, the man developed Bell's palsy. He was tested, found to be positive for *Borrelia burgdorferi,* and diagnosed with Lyme disease. The infection would most likely have been missed had the patient not developed Bell's palsy – a symptom that only nine percent of Lyme disease patients exhibited in the surveillance database of the Centers for Disease Control and Prevention.[166]

This case reminds clinicians of the need to evaluate for other co-infections for atypical presentations and a poor response. In fact, Zaiem and colleagues counsel, "Co-infection with *Borrelia* should be considered in patients with atypical presentation or with a poor response to proper therapy."[166]

"Physicians should consider use of tests designed to diagnose babesiosis and HGE in patients with Lyme disease who experience a prolonged flu-like illness that fails to respond to appropriate antimicrobial therapy,"[119] according to Krause and colleagues. Transverse myelitis[167] and a fatal pancarditis[118] are examples of poor outcomes in patients with both Lyme disease and babesiosis.

The importance of providing follow-up evaluations with patients treated for tick-borne diseases cannot be overstated. Gathering detailed and thorough medical histories is equally as critical because factors not considered important by the patient may impact disease presentation. For instance, Lyme patients may have taken antibiotics prior to their evaluation that could abrogate their immune response.[168-177]

PSYCHIATRIC PRESENTATIONS DELAY LYME DISEASE DIAGNOSIS

Dr. Brian Fallon and colleagues describe a series of patients in 1994 who were thought to suffer from psychiatric illnesses,[18] when, in fact, they had undiagnosed Lyme disease.

The patients were initially presumed to suffer from "paranoia, dementia, schizophrenia, bipolar disorder, panic attacks, major depression, anorexia nervosa, or obsessive-compulsive disorder."[18] Their Lyme disease was overlooked for an average of two years.

Fallon from the Department of Psychiatry, Columbia University Medical Center, and the Lyme Disease Research Program, New York, New York highlighted the difficulty of recognizing Lyme disease in patients with psychiatric manifestations.[178]

"Inattention and poor mental tracking are common features of Lyme encephalopathy in both children and adults. Although impulsivity and hyperactivity may be seen, more often children with Lyme-induced ADHD meet criteria for only the inattention subtype."[178]

"The depression associated with the earlier encephalitic phase of neurologic Lyme disease is characterized by marked irritability and mood lability. Later, in the setting of encephalopathy, the depression is often more mild, characterized primarily by anhedonia, low energy, hopelessness regarding the future, and a diminished sex drive."[178]

Fallon reminded the reader of the need to recognize neuropsychiatric manifestations of Lyme disease. "It has been dubbed "The New Great Imitator" [by Pachner[179]] because, like another spirochetal illness neurosyphilis-the original Great Imitator, Lyme disease has a vast array of multisystem manifestations, including neuropsychiatric ones." Fallon adds, "These three cases demonstrate that patients with Lyme disease may have variable neuropsychiatric presentations, equivocal or negative serologic test results, incomplete treatment response and subsequent relapses."

COULD CHIKUNGUNYA VIRUS SYMPTOMS MIMIC LYME DISEASE?

The Chikungunya virus, which is transmitted by mosquitoes, is posing a real threat to residents of the United States, particularly those living in Florida and the southern states, where the first locally transmitted cases begin to appear.

Chikungunya virus symptoms normally develop three to five days after an infected mosquito bites a person. The virus can cause flu-like symptoms, including fevers, headaches, joint pain, muscle aches, nausea, rashes, and malaise. Those are the same symptoms seen with Lyme disease.

Not all mosquitoes carry the disease. The two types that can transmit Chikungunya virus, *Aedes aegypti* and *Aedes albopictus,* are found in only certain regions of the United States.

A study published in the January 2015 issue of *Arthritis and Rheumatology* raised concerns that "Chikungunya viral arthritis could mimic seronegative rheumatoid arthritis."[180] Miner and colleagues point out the difficulties in making an accurate diagnosis of the Chikungunya virus. Its manifestations are similar to those of rheumatic diseases. And serological testing is only available through the Centers for Disease Control and Prevention, several state health departments, and one commercial laboratory.

The study describes persistent symmetric polyarthritis in people who had traveled to Haiti during a Chikungunya virus outbreak in June 2014. Eight out of the 10 individuals with Chikungunya virus were referred to a St Louis, Mo., rheumatology clinic, where they presented with persistent symmetric polyarthritis. The patients had morning stiffness and chronic arthritis primarily affecting the wrists, hands, ankles, and feet. The chronic arthritis consisted of joint swelling rather than joint destruction. Two of the patients had difficulty walking because of pain in their feet or ankles.

The Chikungunya virus has no preventive vaccines and no treatments other than pain management. The study found that neither naproxen nor acetaminophen was very helpful in alleviating pain. And prednisone (20 mg by mouth daily) failed in one patient because it exacerbated her joint pain and raised a "concern that there could still be a live virus within the joints."[180]

Miner and colleagues remind rheumatologists to consider Chikungunya virus infection when evaluating patients with new symmetric polyarthritis. It would be reasonable to also consider Lyme disease when patients present with new symmetric or asymmetric polyarthritis.

DOCTORS TRY TO MAKE CASE FOR MEDICALLY UNEXPLAINED SYMPTOMS

Shapiro and colleagues have tried to argue that chronically ill children suspected of having Lyme disease were instead suffering from medically unexplained symptoms (MUS).[181] He summarized his findings in a video during the 2014 Pediatric Academic Societies Annual Meeting in Vancouver, Canada.[181]

The term MUS has been used in patients who have significant symptoms but no known physical disease.[1] MUS has been assumed to be a psychiatric diagnosis, and treatment has been dominated by talk therapies.[182] Unigwe and colleagues wrote that "persons with medically unexplained symptoms are often not perceived as having chronic, enduring, mental and physical illness."[182]

The most common symptom attributed to MUS is pain, including diffuse myalgia, arthralgia, low-back pain, headache, and dysuria.[183] Other symptoms include fatigue, insomnia, tinnitus, atypical facial pain, chest pain, palpitations, dyspnea, bloating, nausea, abdominal discomfort, constipation, diarrhea, chronic pelvic pain, dyspareunia, vulvodynia, dysmenorrhea, pseudoseizures, dizziness, and weakness.[183] The term also has been applied to patients with overlapping clusters of symptoms such as irritable bowel syndrome, fibromyalgia, and chronic fatigue.

According to Shapiro and colleagues, Yale Medical Center's pediatric infectious disease clinic found that more than half of the referrals to his clinic were for patients suspected of having Lyme disease. However, Shapiro concluded that 80 percent to 90 percent of those patients were deemed to not have "active" Lyme disease. Instead, he argued they suffered from MUS.

Here are some of Shapiro's descriptions of feedback from families he'd consulted with at his clinic:

- Nearly half of the parents were not happy with the results of the consult visit.
- Nearly half [of the patients] received additional treatment for these ongoing symptoms.
- More than half sought help from providers other than the clinic and their primary care physicians.

The authors did not mention whether he informed parents that there is no test to confirm MUS. Neither did he mention whether he informed parents that there is no clear treatment for MUS.

It's difficult to understand jumping to a diagnosis of MUS in children in the absence of a reliable test or treatment. Careful attention, including consulting with several medical specialists, should be given to this population to make sure that a correct diagnosis is made. It is reasonable to research every avenue that might improve a child's health and quality of life.

BIOLOGICAL EXPLANATIONS MIGHT REDUCE CLINICIANS' EMPATHY

Patients suffering with an illness often turn to their doctors for empathy. This is particularly true for those people living with chronic, often debilitating, symptoms. An understanding practitioner can play an important role in guiding a patient back to health and improving clinical outcomes.

Yet according to a study published in 2014 in the *Proceedings of the National Academy of Sciences*,[184] mental health clinicians may actually be less likely to show empathy toward their patients if there are underlying biological causes of the illness.

The authors "tested the effects of biological explanations among mental health clinicians, specifically examining their empathy toward patients," and found that biological explanations significantly reduced clinicians' empathy. "This is alarming because clinicians' empathy is important for the therapeutic alliance between mental health providers and patients and significantly predicts positive clinical outcomes," the authors point out.[184]

Lyme disease patients need their doctors' understanding, particularly if the disease becomes chronic. The National Institutes of Health

(NIH) trials validated the severity of the illness, even years after patients underwent their initial course of antibiotics.[17,20,73]

Patients who are chronically ill and trying to cope with complications of Lyme disease don't feel empathy when they hear a doctor say that chronic Lyme disease does not exist and any symptoms are nothing more than the aches and pains of daily living.

COULD A PATIENT DIAGNOSED WITH FIBROMYALGIA INSTEAD HAVE LYME DISEASE?

Treatment for fibromyalgia has been somewhat discouraging. Studies have found that serotonin-norepinephrine reuptake inhibitors duloxetine (Cymbalta)[185] and milnacipranz (Savella)[186] were only 30 percent and 50 percent more effective, respectively, than a placebo in reducing the pain of fibromyalgia.

A meta-analysis of 3,808 fibromyalgia patients found that pregabalin (Lyrica), an anticonvulsant drug used for neuropathic pain, also was effective with only a minority of patients achieving moderate or substantial pain relief, [187] as reported by Staube and colleagues from the Department of Occupational and Social Medicine, University of Göttingen, Germany. It has not been established whether these treatments would be effective for other manifestations of fibromyalgia, including fatigue, insomnia, and cognitive and affective symptoms.

If a fibromyalgia patient is not getting better, is it possible that the patient might, in fact, have Lyme disease? The two medical conditions share similar symptoms, making an accurate diagnosis challenging. Consider the following:

- The most common symptoms of fibromyalgia, including fatigue, insomnia, and cognitive and affective presentations,[188] are commonplace in Lyme disease.
- The trigger points described in fibromyalgia[189] are typically referred to as synovitis,[5,190,191] bursitis,[192] and sacroiliitis in Lyme disease.
- There is no laboratory test to confirm fibromyalgia, just as there are no reliable laboratory tests to rule out Lyme.

Patients also might suffer from a combination of both fibromyalgia and Lyme disease. In one study, 4 out of 27 individuals (15 percent) in a chronic neurologic Lyme disease series also presented with fibromyalgia.[16] Three of 25 patients (12 percent) with active Lyme disease who were being seen in a rheumatology-based Lyme disease clinic were also diagnosed with fibromyalgia.[193]

SECTION VIII. CONFLICTS IN THE MEDICAL COMMUNITY

*A*s if the challenges of diagnosing and treating Lyme disease weren't enough, some medical professionals continue to ignore or minimize its existence. They insist that chronic Lyme disease is a myth, and that any case of Lyme or related tick-borne disease can be successfully treated with a single short course of antibiotics. Just as diagnosis and treatment of this complex disease depends on good communication between doctor and patient, resolving conflicts in the medical community demands better dialogue between doctor and doctor.

GUIDELINES SHOULD NOT CONSTRAIN CLINICAL JUDGMENT

The guidelines of the International Lyme and Associated Diseases Society (ILADS) place a high value on the ability of the clinician to exercise clinical judgment.[69] According to the ILADS panel, guidelines should not constrain the treating practitioner from exercising clinical judgment in the absence of strong and compelling evidence to the contrary.

The following points are cited directly from the ILADS guidelines:

- It is reasonable to start with dosages examined in clinical trials, but clinicians may decide to adjust dosages in individual patients with the goal of improving outcomes by achieving adequate drug levels in all infected tissues.
- If the initial course of antibiotic retreatment does not produce a complete response, clinicians should consider various options. Patients who had an incomplete response with one agent may be responsive to another; thus, switching agents may prove successful.
- Treatment regimens may employ either a sole agent or combination of antibiotics, depending on which mechanisms

of persistence the clinician is attempting to thwart. The delivery method – oral, intravenous (IV), or intramuscular (IM) – is dependent on the agents selected, disease severity, and patient preferences.

The ILADS guidelines discuss a range of antibiotics, including oral amoxicillin, phenoxymethyl penicillin, tetracycline, and macrolide classes; metronidazole; IV ceftriaxone, cefotaxime, and penicillin; and IM benzathine penicillin. The guidelines recommend that clinicians advise patients to take probiotics daily while on antibiotic therapy to reduce the risk of *C. difficile* colitis and antibiotic-associated diarrhea.

GUIDELINES ARE TOO RESTRICTIVE FOR DOCTORS IN PRACTICE

According to the 2006 evidenced-based guidelines of the Infectious Disease Society of America (IDSA), patients only need a single, 200-mg dose of Doxycycline for a known tick bite; or, a single, 10-to-21 days of antibiotics for Lyme disease. The only exception is adding 30 days of antibiotics if the patient has been diagnosed with Lyme arthritis.[70]

The IDSA guidelines, however, have been questioned by many physicians treating Lyme disease patients. The International Lyme and Associated Diseases Society (ILADS), using GRADE assessment for its evidence-based treatment guidelines, found that the IDSA treatment protocols are of very low quality because of limitations in trial designs, imprecise findings, outcome inconsistencies, and the inability to generalize trial findings.[69]

For example, it is impossible to state a meaningful success rate for the IDSA recommendation of a single 200-mg dose of doxycycline because the sole trial of that regimen used an inadequate observation period and had no validated surrogate end point.

Moreover, the success rate for a 21-day treatment of an erythema migrans rash was no better than 52.2 percent to 84.4 percent using an Intent-to-Treat analysis.

Research is needed to better define the disease process, identify variables associated with poor outcomes, and establish the most effective therapeutic regimens for known tick bites, erythema migrans rashes, and persistent disease. An optimal treatment regimen for these conditions has not yet been determined.

For now, the IDSA guidelines for treating Lyme disease can be too restrictive for doctors in practice. Given the number of clinical variables that must be managed and the many differences within the patient population, clinical judgment is crucial to providing patient-centered care.

PATIENTS SHOULD BE INFORMED OF CONFLICTING TREATMENT GUIDELINES

Two medical societies offer guidelines for the treatment of Lyme disease — the Infectious Diseases Society of America (IDSA) and the International Lyme and Associated Diseases Society (ILADS).

But doctors remain in limbo as discussions between the two societies stall.

At least 300,000 new cases of Lyme disease show up in doctors' offices throughout the country each year, and that number will grow. It would be reasonable for physicians to inform patients of both the 2006 IDSA[194] and the 2014 ILADS[195] treatment guidelines.

TIME TO DESIGNATE LYME DISEASE AS A PANDEMIC?

*L*yme disease has been referred to as hyperendemic in some areas. Hyperendemic is defined as "exhibiting a high and continued incidence." But today, Lyme disease hardly fits that definition.

So, is it time to designate Lyme disease as a pandemic?

Pandemic is defined as an outbreak of a disease that occurs over a wide geographic area and affects an exceptionally high proportion of the population.[196] Recently published reviews have described the worldwide distribution of Lyme disease and other tick-borne illnesses.[58] Thirty percent of the residents sampled in Connecticut had received treatment for a tick-transmitted illness, while 50 percent reported another family member having had a tick-borne disease.[197]

Morens and colleagues described eight basic characteristics that apply to all or almost all pandemics in the *Journal of Infectious Diseases*.[198]

1. wide geographic extension
2. disease movement
3. high attack rates and explosiveness

4. minimal population immunity
5. novelty
6. infectiousness
7. contagiousness
8. severity

Lyme disease meets those eight characteristics.[198] The disease is distributed worldwide, is moved long distances by birds, has a high attack rate and explosive spread, offers minimal immunity, has novelty, can lead to a wide range of chronic manifestations not previously described, is transmitted by a vector, and can lead to severe illness.[17,20]

Designating a medical condition as pandemic allows physicians, scientists, and public health officials to justify funding and commitment of resources. Other diseases designated pandemic include acute hemorrhagic conjunctivitis (AHC), acquired immune deficiency syndrome (AIDS), cholera, dengue, influenza, obesity, plague, severe acute respiratory syndrome (SARS), scabies, and West Nile disease.

It's time for Lyme disease to be designated as a pandemic. This reclassification might then empower physicians, scientists, and public health officials with a stronger argument to justify increased funding and commitment of resources to more aggressively study the disease.

RECOMMENDATIONS IGNORE CHRONIC MANIFESTATIONS OF LYME DISEASE

A review of treatment recommendations in a 2016 issue of the *Journal of the American Medical Association (JAMA)* focused on early Lyme disease rather than chronic manifestations of tick-borne illness.[199]

"Multiple trials have shown efficacy for a 10-day course of oral doxycycline for treatment of erythema migrans and for a 14-day course for treatment of early neurologic Lyme disease in ambulatory patients," the review concludes.[199] Furthermore, "Evidence indicates that a 10-day course of oral doxycycline is effective for HGA [human granulocytic anaplasmosis] and that a 7- to 10-day course of azithromycin plus atovaquone is effective for mild babesiosis."[199]

The review overlooks the poor outcomes of treating early Lyme disease using an Intent-to-Treat analysis in the 2014 guidelines of the International Lyme and Associated Diseases (ILADS) guidelines. Intent-to-Treat analyses are thought to better represent clinical realities, where patients may inadvertently or purposefully change or abandon treatment.

The Intent-to-Treat analysis review by ILADS demonstrates low success rates even for patients treated at the time of an erythema migrans rash. The success rates varied from 52 percent to 78 percent a year after treatment.[69]

The *JAMA* review[199] also overlooked chronic manifestations beyond a year of treatment, including chronic neurologic Lyme disease,[16] Lyme encephalopathy,[17,68] post Lyme disease,[73] post-treatment Lyme disease syndrome,[19] and persistent symptoms with a history of Lyme disease.[124]

MEDICINE'S WORST KEPT SECRET: CHRONIC MANIFESTATIONS OF LYME DISEASE EXIST

Some doctors have interpreted the Infectious Diseases Society of America (IDSA) guidelines to mean there are no chronic manifestations of Lyme disease, and any lingering symptoms are nothing more than the aches and pains of daily living.[70]

Those conclusions overlook years of study published by leading university researchers.

- Twenty-seven Lyme disease patients were ill up to 14 years with Lyme encephalopathy and Lyme neuropathy after antibiotic treatment.[16]
- Thirty-four percent of a population-based, retrospective cohort were ill an average of 6.2 years after antibiotic treatment.[77]
- Sixty-two percent of a retrospective evaluation of 215 Lyme disease patients from Westchester County, N.Y., remained ill an average of 3.2 years after antibiotic treatment.[76]
- Fifty-seven percent of 30 adults with Lyme neuroborreliosis remained ill years after treatment at the Medical Center, University of Freiburg.[135]

- In a meta-analysis study, 504 patients treated for Lyme disease had more fatigue, musculoskeletal pain, and neurocognitive difficulties than 530 controls.[200]
- The National Institutes of Health (NIH) sponsored two trials that enrolled 78 patients who were seropositive for IgG antibodies and 51 patients who were not. On average, the seropositive patients had persistent symptoms 4.7 years after onset of their illness.[124]
- Also in an NIH-sponsored trial, 55 patients with Lyme disease had persistent severe fatigue six or more months after antibiotic therapy.[73]
- In an NIH trial of Lyme encephalopathy, 37 patients with at least three weeks of prior IV antibiotics and current positive IgG western blot had objective memory impairment.
- Of 63 patients treated with three weeks of doxycycline in a Johns Hopkins study, 36 percent reported new-onset fatigue, 20 percent reported widespread pain, and 45 percent reported neurocognitive difficulties six months after treatment.[19]

It's time for medicine to accept that chronic manifestations of Lyme disease exist, and the lingering symptoms can be serious.[70]

THE MEDICAL COMMUNITY FORCED OUT OF ITS COMFORT ZONE

"The medical community has been collectively forced out of its comfort zone on Lyme disease by increasing evidence of the complexity of this multisystem disease,"[201] insists Borgermans and colleagues, Vrije Universiteit, Brussels.[201] The researchers further note, "We need more national and international debates on Lyme disease, complemented by a solid research agenda and a focus on cutting edge biological technologies," Borgermans and colleagues say.

"Most patients will present to family physicians, who often have few subsequent resources when the initial treatment proves unsuccessful,"[201] they wrote in the December 2015 issue of the *British Medical Journal*.

Borgermans and colleagues recommend discussions include family doctors, who could be instrumental in advancing the dialogue. "Family physicians can act as important partners alongside infectious disease specialists and others to drive this debate forward."

Borgermans and colleagues' editorial recounts the following issues they raised two years earlier in the *International Journal of Family Medicine* and have yet to be resolved.

- range of clinical presentations, including between sexes
- diagnostic criteria and tools
- treatments and their efficacy
- transmission modes and vectors
- role of co-infections
- uncertainty over clinical definition of chronic Lyme disease and whether detection of active infection is essential
- whether and for how long the pathogen can persist
- role of psychoneuroimmunology, host-pathogen interactions, and autoimmunity in residual or persisting antigens
- role of toxins or other bacterial products in symptoms and signs
- contribution of environmental factors[202]

Borgermans and colleagues also point out the consequences of putting off a dialogue, citing the medical community's long delay in recognizing the role *Helicobacter pylori* played in gastric disease. This demonstrates the "consequences of ignoring findings that contradict our current beliefs about a disease."[201]

The editorial concludes with an urgent call for action. "In an era where patient centered care is considered the cornerstone of high quality and integrated medicine, we cannot allow ourselves to repeat past mistakes at our patients' expense. The suffering of many affected patients obliges us to learn more about this disease."[201]

'FAKE NEWS' CHARGES DO NOT GIVE PROFESSIONALS CREDIT

*C*ountless professionals—from physicians to researchers and citizen scientists—have been working earnestly to try and understand Lyme disease. And, the Lyme disease professional community can and should take credit for and celebrate some of the following findings:

1. Dr. Alan Steere and colleagues described a cluster of adolescents and adults in Lyme, Conn., suffering from what was named Lyme disease rather than juvenile rheumatoid arthritis.[5]
2. Dr. William Burgdorfer and colleagues discovered *Borrelia burgdorferi* in the midgut of *Ixodes scapularis* ticks.[6]
3. Dr. James Krause and colleagues discovered *Babesia microti* in the same ticks.[60]
4. Dr. Eric Logigian and colleagues described chronic neurologic Lyme and Lyme encephalopathy in patients despite antibiotic treatment.[16]

Yet, these discoveries, and many more which readers of this book have already encountered, are severely diminished (or nearly ignored) when other physicians level charges that Lyme disease is not a problem, but rather the problem is "fake research," "fake blood cultures," "fake diagnoses," and "fake laboratory research." [203]

In fact, authors Shapiro, Baker and Wormser go so far as to suggest legislators stop passing laws to protect physicians who treat Lyme disease, arguing such laws make "it difficult for medical review boards to safeguard public health by disciplining those who put patients at risk."

If the medical community truly wishes to broaden its knowledge of Lyme disease, it would be more reasonable to give credit to the Lyme disease community that has worked tirelessly to understand this complex disease, as opposed to dismissing findings as baseless. Articles that claim Lyme disease patients, advocates, and professionals are pushing "fake news" do little to further our knowledge of Lyme disease and its co-infections

SHARED DECISION-MAKING APPROACH TO PATIENT-CENTERED MEDICINE

In recent years, there's been a transformation, to some degree, within the medical establishment regarding the physician-patient relationship. Healthcare institutions have been actively trying to change the way physicians and patients interact with one another, using a shared decision-making approach to achieve patient-centered medicine.

The goal is to move away from a model of care where the doctor is the sole voice with treatment decisions toward a patient-centered practice that fully involves the patient in each decision at every stage of care. Slowly but steadily, the medical community has responded, adopting a shared decision-making process with a broad range of illnesses, including prostate cancer, diabetes, and even asthma.

Penn State Medical College recently began training its medical students on patient-centered medicine.[204]

"While clinicians know information about the disease, tests, and treatments, the patient knows information about their body, their circumstances, their goals for life and healthcare," according to a 2015 study.[205]

Shared decision-making empowers patients, giving them a voice in treatment choices. The International Lyme and Associated Diseases Society's evidence-based treatment guidelines encourage shared decision-making to improve outcomes for patients with complications of Lyme disease.[69]

Clinicians must embrace this open approach when treating Lyme disease patients. Empowering patients in the decision making process invests them in the time and compliance it takes to manage and potentially cure the disease or diseases left by a tick bite. And, until researchers and medicine find a consistent treatment approach to these infections which work for the majority of patients, patients must keep track of their treatment should they need to change physicians.

CLINICIANS URGED TO TAILOR THERAPY BASED ON THE PATIENT'S RESPONSE

The Infectious Diseases Society of America (IDSA) has concluded that the evidence is so overwhelming strong in supporting its guidelines that treating physicians do not need to tailor therapy based on a patient's response. [70]

The IDSA guidelines advise the following:

- a one-time 200 mg dose of doxycycline for a tick bite
- 10 to 21 days of antibiotics for an erythema migrans rash
- retreatment for a month for Lyme arthritis only

The International Lyme and Associated Diseases Society (ILADS) concluded that the evidence base for these three IDSA recommendations to be of low or very low quality in the treatment of Lyme disease.[69] Instead, ILADS supports individualized risk/benefit assessments and shared decision-making.

Examples taken from the ILADS guidelines include the following:

- Shared decision-making takes into account the best scientific evidence available, clinical expertise, and the role of the

patient's values and preferences in deciding among available treatment options.
- The panel recognizes that there is a need for clinicians, in the context of shared medical decision-making, to engage in a risk/benefit assessment that reflects the individual values of each patient.
- Patients vary considerably in their tolerance for risk and in what they regard as a valuable benefit. Patients may also tolerate more risk when they have severe presentations of disease or when there are no other treatment options available.
- Given what readers have learned from the last conversation about the importance of shared decision-making, it's hard to understand why the IDSA would suggest doctors ignore how patients are responding to treatment. How should a doctor respond to a patient who self-reports: *I don't feel any better?*

DOCTORS SHOULD NOT BE IMPATIENT OR DISMISSIVE

Lantos and colleagues at Duke University Medical Center offer suggestions to physicians on how to manage patients complaining of chronic Lyme disease in the June 2015 issue of *Infectious Disease Clinics of North America.*[206]

"Even if chronic Lyme disease lacks biological legitimacy, its importance as a phenomenon can be monumental to the individual patient," say the authors. "Many have undergone frustrating, expensive, and ultimately fruitless medical evaluations. And many have become quite disaffected with a medical system that has failed to provide answers."[206]

Lantos and colleagues offer the following advice:

- First, "The physician needs to suppress preconceptions or biases about such patients."[206]
- Second, "The process of clinical information gathering in medicine is no different in the context of chronic Lyme disease, even if much discussion is centered on chronic Lyme disease."[206]
- And lastly, "It is of utmost importance to not seem to be

impatient, dismissive, or rushed. Many patients who seek care for chronic Lyme disease already have accumulated frustration. Each patient's clinical story and personal history is unique and valid, even if one concludes that they do not have Lyme disease."[206]

This advice might also be used to suppress preconceptions that chronic manifestations of Lyme disease do not exist, based on the 2006 guidelines of the Infectious Diseases Society of America.[70] It also might help to avoid the accumulated frustration with expensive and ultimately fruitless medical evaluations for any condition but Lyme disease.

CDC TAKES SWIFT AND AGGRESSIVE ACTION ON THE ZIKA OUTBREAK

Although Lyme disease and the Zika virus are transmitted by different types of vectors, both illnesses can cause severe, long-term health damage and are of enormous concern to the public. The response by the Centers for Disease Control and Prevention (CDC) to each threat, however, has been decidedly different.

The CDC responded to the Zika outbreak with swift and aggressive action; while patients suffering from Lyme disease and other co-infections continue to wait for the CDC to declare tick infections a public health problem.

"On Jan. 22, 2016, the CDC activated its Emergency Operations Center to respond to outbreaks of Zika occurring in the Americas and increased reports of birth defects and Guillain-Barré syndrome in areas affected by Zika," wrote the CDC in a message posted on its website. [207]

Two weeks later, on Feb. 8, 2016, the CDC elevated its Emergency Operations Center activation to Level 1, the highest level.[207]

The Zika virus is spread primarily by the *Aedes aegypti* mosquito; the insect is best-known as the vector for viruses that cause yellow fever, dengue, and Chikungunya. In a February 2016 interview with National Public Radio (NPR), Marten Edwards, Ph.D., a research entomologist at Muhlenberg College in Allentown, Pa., described the mosquito capturing everyone's attention.

"The stomach of the *Aedes aegypti* is a fertile place for the Zika virus to reproduce. This doesn't happen in the vast majority of mosquitoes," Edwards said. "So that's what makes the *Aedes aegypti* unusual."[208]

He continued, "The mosquito's feeding habits are another boon for viral spreading. In general, female mosquitoes bite people or other warm-blooded creatures because they need the blood to hatch their eggs. Most mosquitoes get some blood in one bite and get on with reproduction. But *Aedes aegypti* is what's known as a 'sip feeder.' It takes lots of little sips of blood from lots of people. So once an *Aedes aegypti* mosquito is infected with a virus, it's able to spread it multiple times in its two- to four-week life."[208]

Edwards explained, "It's a tricky mosquito to control. It doesn't bite at night like the mosquitoes that transmit malaria, so bed nets are not necessarily useful. They rest both inside and outside houses, so there's not an easy way to target the adult mosquito [with pesticide]."[208]

Studying the habits of insects like *Aedes aegypti* mosquitoes, and arthropods like *Ixodes scapularis* begin to lead scientists to potential ways to control infections and the spread of diseases like the Zika virus and Lyme disease.

The CDC mission statement says, "Whether diseases start at home or abroad, are chronic or acute, curable or preventable, human error or deliberate attack, CDC fights disease and supports communities and citizens to do the same." [209] However in the cases of Zika and Lyme disease, the CDC's response was not equal or consistent.

CENTER YET TO SEE A LYME ENCEPHALOPATHY CASE

Some physicians have yet to see Lyme encephalopathy or axonal neuropathy cases, according to a review article in *Wien Klin Wochenschr*. "We have never seen the poorly defined entity referred to as Lyme encephalopathy and question its existence,"[210] according to Wormser and colleagues from ghd Lyme Disease Diagnostic Center, Division of Infectious Diseases, New York Medical College, Valhalla, N.Y.

Other physicians have seen many Lyme encephalopathy cases, and the condition has been described in numerous published reports. Dr. Allen Steere, best known for discovering Lyme disease, was one of the authors that described Lyme encephalopathy in 1990.[5] "Twenty four of 27 chronic Lyme disease patients presented with a mild encephalopathy that began 1 month to 14 years after the onset of the disease and was characterized by memory loss, mood changes, and sleep disturbances."

Lyme encephalopathy was again described both in the 1990 *Journal of Infectious Diseases*[68] and the 2009 National Institutes of Health-sponsored trial published in *Neurology*.[17]

How could the center in Valhalla, N.Y., have yet to see a Lyme encephalopathy case?

The answer could be that the center typically sees individuals in the acute phase of the disease. The center is usually open for just a couple hours a day during the summer months.[210]

It would be reasonable to acknowledge that other physicians and centers have described Lyme encephalopathy or axonal neuropathy.

ONE TRIAL AND THREE JOURNAL ARTICLES, YET THE RESEARCHER FAILED TO RECOGNIZE THE COMPLICATIONS OF LYME DISEASE.

When does research become a bully pulpit and a cudgel? When the researcher wants to prove his or her point (as opposed to finding an answer to a question) and one's like-minded colleagues cite an erroneous conclusion over and over.

In 2015, Gary Wormser, MD and colleagues published three articles, in three different journals, concluding the number of patients with Lyme who suffer continued bouts of fatigue and fibromyalgia, are no different from the number of people in the general population who suffer from the same symptoms.

The narrative from Wormser and colleagues began with the assertion that the risk of fibromyalgia, chronic fatigue, and a diminished quality of life was described by patients as negligible 11 to 20 years after treatment for an erythema migrans rash. The quality of life for 100 patients was "virtually identical" to the general population 11 to 20 years after diagnosis, according to a study.[211]

In a different reporting of the same clinical trial, the researchers noted only one out of the 100 patients (1 percent) who remained in their study developed fibromyalgia; and that patient developed it 19 years after the Lyme disease diagnosis – suggesting there was no correlation.[212]

In a third journal article, the researchers wrote, only nine patients (9 percent) complained of severe fatigue.[213] So, the conclusion was, "our study has demonstrated that the long-term health-related quality of life of patients with culture-confirmed early Lyme disease, when assessed by the SF-36 survey, is on average similar to that of the general United States population."[211]

However, upon further reflection, the trial overlooked previous research identifying the complications of Lyme disease, and failed to identify the reason more than half of the enrolled subjects dropped from the study.

The incidence of fibromyalgia and chronic fatigue was evident more than 14 years after treatment, when 60 percent of the 283 patients who entered the study were already lost to follow-up. Also, the study did not include other, previously identified, complications of Lyme disease, including chronic neurologic Lyme[16] and Lyme encephalopathy.[68]

Consequently, other authors have cited the study by Wormers and his colleagues in an effort to dismiss the risk of complications of Lyme disease.[206,214] "This study should help suppress concerns that the effects of early Lyme disease are likely to cause lifelong debilitation,"[214] according to Auwaerter and colleagues from the Johns Hopkins University School of Medicine.

"Only 1 of 100 patients treated for culture-confirmed Lyme disease developed fibromyalgia during the subsequent 11 to 20 years,"[206] reported Lantos and others from the Division of General Internal Medicine, and Division of Pediatric Infectious Diseases at Duke University Medical Center.

And so, the message gets cited over and over; read by thousands of medical professionals who take the study results at face value, and don't necessarily examine the flaws in the details or design.

Consequently, the findings of Wormser et.al. cannot be generalized to actual practice because of the severe limitations of the study. In real life, physicians need to address the health of Lyme disease patients who are not treated at the time of the rash. They also need to document and pay close attention to those with continued symptoms and complaints.

NEITHER TWO NOR 14 WEEKS OF ANTIBIOTICS EFFECTIVE IN NETHERLANDS TRIAL

Berende and colleagues reported poor outcomes in a European trial in which 280 Lyme patients with persistent symptoms were treated for a total of fourteen weeks in a randomized, double-blind study.[125]

The study began with everyone in the study receiving antibiotics for two weeks. "All the patients received treatment with 2000 mg of open-label intravenous ceftriaxone daily for 14 days," the researchers noted in a study published in *The New England Journal of Medicine*.[125]

Patients were then divided into three groups in order to complete the trial. Over the remaining 12 weeks, patients received oral courses of either doxycycline and a placebo twice daily; clarithromycin–hydroxychloroquine twice daily; or a placebo dose.

Ninety-eight of their patients with persistent Lyme disease symptoms demonstrated only a slight improvement in their quality of life following a two-week course of intravenous ceftriaxone. The patients' physical-component summary score (a score which measures quality of life) rose by only 3 points. And even that slight change in the quality of life, scores from those Lyme patients remained below that of cancer and heart-attack patients, and well below the normal of 50 for the general population.

The same 98 patients received 12 additional weeks of antibiotics; and again, the physical-component summary score did not significantly improve.

There are several reasons why both short-and-long term therapies failed:

- The patients had failed two previous treatments.
- The patients had been ill for 2.7 years prior to the trial.
- Their quality of life remained poor after the trial.
- They were not evaluated for co-infections (e.g., Babesia).

Several other treatment options were not discussed for the 98 patients:

- Consider treating all patients with more than two weeks of intravenous ceftriaxone.
- Consider treating patients sooner than the 2.7 years after onset of illness described in the trial.
- Consider evaluation and treatment for co-infections (e.g., Babesia).
- Consider individualized therapy for each patient until quality of life returns to normal.

SECTION IX. TREATMENT OPTIONS

Researchers continue to seek a better understanding of just how Lyme disease and its co-infections damage the body in an effort to design better treatment protocols. These researchers especially want to know why some patients suffer chronic symptoms despite having treatment for a tick bite. The conversations which follow look at laboratory studies designed to understand how Lyme bacteria respond at a cellular level to unusual combinations of drugs. There are also studies which aim to help develop retreatment protocols for the chronic neurologic diseases Lyme patients wrestle with. Finally, researchers continue to examine treatment options in an effort to find the most effective ways to manage chronic Lyme disease.

ILADS GUIDELINES HAVE BEEN DISSEMINATED AND IMPLEMENTED

The Infectious Diseases Society of America (IDSA) had been criticized by both physicians and patients for not recognizing the existence and severity of chronic manifestations of Lyme disease in their 2006 guidelines.[70] In response to what it considered a significant oversight, the International Lyme and Associated Diseases Society (ILADS) published guidelines in 2014 which identified and addressed the existence and severity of chronic manifestations of Lyme disease.[69]

The ILADS guidelines were developed using a tool called the Grading of Recommendations Assessment, Development, and Evaluation, or GRADE. The GRADE system is a methodology which provides a way to examine and assess research in an effort to assure three basic goals are met when developing treatment protocols.

First, GRADE insures research methods used to study treatment plans are strong and precise. Secondly, studies must have a strong and direct effect on the patient population in a study. And finally, GRADE standards require that there are few downsides to therapy.[215] Thus, GRADE considers the balance between the benefits and harm of various interventions, confidence in the estimates of effects, patient preferences and values, and resource use[69]

The ILADS guidelines were peer reviewed and published in the open-accessed journal *Expert Review of Anti-Infective Therapy*[195] and accepted by the National Guideline Clearing House.[216] ILADS guidelines were presented at professional conferences and incorporated into the ILADS physician training program.[217]

The ILADS evidence-based guidelines have ranked in the top five percent of all research articles, as scored by Altmetrics, with more than 178,152 downloads as of May 2017. Altmetrics is a measure of the reach and influence of research publications.[218]

And there's evidence that physicians are implementing recommendations described in the ILADS guidelines.

- In 2011, 50 percent of New England physicians surveyed said they believed "prolonged treatment [with antibiotics] was sometimes useful," and an estimated 25 percent thought it was "always useful,"[219] according to Macauda and colleagues from the Department of Health Promotion, Education, and Behavior, Arnold School of Public Health, University of South Carolina, Columbia, S.C.
- In a review of insurance claims data published in 2015, 18 percent of Lyme disease patients were treated for more than five weeks, according to Tseng and colleagues from the Computational Health Informatics Program, Boston Children's Hospital, Boston, Mass.[220]

LINGERING CONCERNS ABOUT THE LYME DISEASE VACCINE

A new, closer look (or meta-analysis) of the recombinant vaccine against Lyme disease by Zhao et. al. failed to address continued lingering concerns about the vaccine's safety and effectiveness in patients.[221] A recombinant vaccine is made by recombining DNA material in an effort to evoke an immune response in a patient.

The vaccine, called LYMErix, was developed by GlaxoSmithKline and approved by the Food and Drug Administration (FDA) on Dec. 21, 1998. The vaccine aims to leverage the role OspA plays in Lyme disease.

OspA is shorthand for Outer Surface Protein A (OspA). The Lyme disease causing bacteria, *B. burgdorferi* is coated with OspA (and several others up to OspF thus far). Researchers believe this OspA coating may play a role in how *B. burgdorferi* survives within the tick gut. OspA may also play a role in disease transmission and the intensity (or virulence) of the disease in a patient.

Here are the concerns about LYMErix which have yet to be adequately addressed.'

- The LYMErix vaccine trial, based on the outer surface protein A (OspA) of *Borrelia burgdorferi*, was 78 percent effective at preventing a culture-confirmed erythema migrans rash.[221]
- The vaccine was only 48 percent effective at preventing what the safety insert from GlaxoSmithKline referred to as "possible Lyme disease."[222] Possible Lyme disease was defined as "a flu-like illness (fever, chills, fatigue, headache, joint or muscle aches) with IgM or IgG Western blot seroconversion, or physician-diagnosed erythema migrans with negative laboratory results."[222]
- The OspA vaccine was minimally effective in subjects vaccinated only twice.[222]
- The efficacy of the OspA vaccine beyond the second year was inconclusive.[223]
- The OspA was not evaluated for the *B. garinii* and *B. afzelii* genospecies described in Europe.[223]
- The vaccine trial did not address whether the OspA vaccine would prevent other complications of Lyme disease, including Lyme encephalopathy or post-treatment Lyme disease syndrome.

The Lyme disease vaccine was removed from the market in 2002. The Centers for Disease Control and Prevention website warns, "Protection provided by this vaccine diminishes over time. Therefore, if you received the Lyme disease vaccine before 2002, you are probably no longer protected against Lyme disease."[224]

An NBC News report summarized concerns with the Lyme disease vaccine. "There once was a human Lyme disease vaccine on the market, but its maker, GlaxoSmithKline, stopped making it after rumors about its safety and multiple lawsuits filed by people claiming it made them sick. The company said it couldn't sell enough doses to make it worthwhile."[225]

The meta-analysis by Zhao and colleagues suggested that a new-generation, multivalent OspA-based Lyme borreliosis vaccine might be more effective against all *B. burgdorferi sensu lato* strains.

In the meantime, it would be helpful if any lingering concerns with the LYMErix vaccine were addressed first.

CASE STUDY: MINNESOTA TRAVELER CONTRACTS B. MIYAMOTOI AND B. BURGDORFERI

*D*octors describe a case of *Borrelia miyamotoi* in a previously healthy 63-year-old American man living in Japan. "He reported being bitten by ticks several times while staying with his family at his summer house in the state of Minnesota in the United States from July 25 to August 9, 2013," according to Oda and colleagues from the Division of Infectious Diseases, Musashino Red Cross Hospital, Japan.[226]

He presented with a 10-day history of malaise, headache, myalgia, and arthralgia following his return to Japan from Minnesota. His evaluation revealed a high fever (39.2° C), erythema migrans, slightly elevated aspartate aminotransferase and alanine aminotransferase levels (39 IU/L and 77 IU/L, respectively), and elevated C-reactive protein level (7.73 mg/dL).

The man was diagnosed with *B. miyamotoi* by seroreactivity to recombinant glycerophosphodiester phosphodiesterase (rGlpQ). "The accuracy of rGlpQ serodiagnosis was originally designated by Schwan and colleagues,[227] and is an alternative method when bacterial DNA is not detected," according to the authors.

He was also diagnosed with Lyme disease based on the erythema migrans rash and three IgM bands: 24 kDa (OspC), 39 kDa (BmpA), and 41 kDa (Fla). The authors did not mention whether they looked for other tick-borne illnesses reported in Minnesota such as Babesia, Ehrlichia, and anaplasmosis.

"This case suggests that *B. miyamotoi* should be considered in febrile travelers returning from the Northeastern and Midwestern regions of the United States," state Oda and colleagues.[226]

The Minnesota traveler gradually improved over 14 days on doxycycline. "Amoxicillin, cefuroxime, and macrolide also may be effective [citing Krause and colleagues[12]]," wrote the authors.[226]

It remains to be seen whether short courses of antibiotics will be effective to prevent complications of *B. miyamotoi* or *B. burgdorferi*. A follow-up report on this patient would be illustrative.

JOHNS HOPKINS STUDY SUPPORTS EARLY RETREATMENT

Many Lyme disease patients continue to suffer for years after antibiotic treatment. For example, patients with chronic neurologic Lyme disease have been ill for up to 14 years.[16] Additionally, other patients suffer continued symptoms such as "fatigue, myalgias, arthralgias without arthritis, dysesthesias or paresthesias, or mood and memory disturbances after the standard courses of antibiotics."[124] Patients enrolling in three National Institutes of Health sponsored trials were ill with chronic symptoms for an average of 4.7 to 9 years.[17,20]

In the *Archives of Clinical Neuropsychology*, Bechtold and colleagues from the Department of Physical Medicine and Rehabilitation, Johns Hopkins University School of Medicine acknowledged a substantial number of patients suffered from severe fatigue, pain, and Post-Treatment Lyme Disease Syndrome (PTLDS) six months after completing a three-week course of antibiotics for an erythema migrans rash.[123] Out of 107 patients, 23 (21 percent) had a high fatigue total score and 33 (31 percent) had a high pain score. Additionally, six of the 107 patients (6 percent) had PTLDS. Only five patients (5 percent) had a high depression total score.

Bechtold et. al. suggest, "Patients with symptoms of pain, fatigue, and depression on standardized instruments can be referred for appropriate behavioral and medicinal interventions to reduce the impact of these symptoms on daily life functioning." The researchers added, "If there is sufficient concern after education and interventions have been applied, then patients can be referred for neuropsychological evaluation."[123]

In fact, Bechtold and colleagues identified eight cases for early retreatment. "Of the 107 cases, eight cases were retreated with antibiotics after the initial 3-week course of doxycycline because there was development of new objective findings (e.g., new neuropathy; five cases) or the EM rash did not fade after initial treatment or new rashes developed in other areas of the body (three cases)," according to Bechtold and colleagues.[123] Only two of the six PTLDS patients were retreated. Most of the cases with severe fatigue and pain were not retreated.

In another study, a group of Hopkins researchers suggest retreatment with antibiotics should be considered when symptoms persist. According to Aucott and colleagues from Johns Hopkins University School of Medicine, "Studies using rodent and primate models have suggested that the persistence of bacteria and/or spirochetal antigens after antibiotic therapy may drive disease,"[130] These researchers also suggest, "The use of short-term antibiotic retreatment in the early, post-treatment phase of Lyme disease has yet to be formally tested, although it may be widely applied in clinical practice."

ANTIBIOTICS EFFECTIVE FOR SOME BUT NOT ALL NEUROLOGIC COMPLICATIONS

When making treatment decisions, doctors often turn to the Cochrane Review, which is described on the Review's website as "a global independent network of researchers, professionals, patients, carers, and people interested in health." Cochrane is comprised of 37,000 contributors from over 130 countries who "work together to produce credible, accessible health information that is free from commercial sponsorship and other conflicts of interest."[228]

An article published in Cochrane by Cadavid and colleagues describes generally favorable outcomes for treating neurologic complications of Lyme disease in Europe. "The majority of people are reported to have good outcomes, and symptoms resolve by 12 months regardless of the antibiotic used. A minority of participants did not improve sufficiently, and some were retreated. These randomized studies provide some evidence that doxycycline, penicillin G, ceftriaxone, and cefotaxime are efficacious in the treatment of European LNB [Lyme neuroborreliosis]."[229]

Doctors may find it surprising that the Cochrane Review failed to identify a single trial on the antibiotic treatment of neurologic complications from Lyme disease in the United States. "We excluded non-randomized and uncontrolled studies. We also excluded single-case reports and case series," explains Cadavid.[229]

As a result, clinicians in the United States have had to rely on research data not included in the Cochrane Review when making treatment decisions for patients with neurologic complications of Lyme disease.

Antibiotic treatment has been effective for some but not all neurologic complications of Lyme diseases.

- In a chronic neurologic Lyme disease case series, 63 percent of patients treated with two weeks of intravenous ceftriaxone improved, 22 percent improved but then relapsed, and 15 percent failed to improve.[16]
- In a Lyme encephalopathy case series, 26 percent of patients treated with four weeks of intravenous ceftriaxone returned to normal, 32 percent greatly improved, 16 percent somewhat improved (5 percent requiring retreatment), and 16 percent dropped out.[68]
- In a trial sponsored by the National Institutes of Health at Columbia School of Medicine, New York, patients treated with 10 weeks of intravenous ceftriaxone saw significant improvement in their fatigue but not in their primary outcome of cognitive function.[17]

The research implications are clear. Patients and their treating physicians would benefit from more rigorous research on treatment options for complications of Lyme disease.

ONE-TIME, SINGLE DOSE OF DOXYCYCLINE FOR A TICK BITE PROBLEM

In a recent review entitled "Lyme Disease: Emergency Department Considerations," the authors recommend using a one-time, single dose of doxycycline for the prophylactic treatment of a tick bite, despite the fact that there has been only one study exploring the effectiveness of such a limited dosage. [230] Prophylactic treatment is, by definition, designed to prevent a disease from taking hold in the body. The review failed to mention that the single dose of doxycycline approach advised by the Infectious Diseases Society of America (IDSA) [70] was based on only one prophylactic study.

There were only nine erythema migrans rashes in the Nadelman prophylactic study in 2001 in the *New England Journal of Medicine*. There was only one rash in the treatment group, compared with eight in the placebo group. The p value was barely significant at 0.04.

The prophylactic trial had several other limitations:

- It was not designed to detect Lyme disease if the erythema migrans rash was absent.

- It was not designed to detect chronic or late manifestations of Lyme disease beyond the six weeks of observation.
- It was not designed to assess whether a single dose of doxycycline might be effective for preventing other tick-borne illnesses, such as *Ehrlichia, Anaplasmosis,* or *A. miyamotoi.*
- The previous three prophylactic trials had failed

The 2014 guidelines of the International Lyme and Associated Diseases Society (ILADS) concluded that the evidence for a single, 200-mg prophylactic treatment with doxycycline was "sparse, coming from a single study with few events, and, thus, imprecise."[69]

ILADS makes the following three recommendations.

- Clinicians should **not** use a single, 200-mg dose of doxycycline for Lyme disease prophylaxis.
- Clinicians should promptly offer antibiotic prophylaxis for known *Ixodes* tick bites in which there is evidence of tick feeding, regardless of the degree of tick engorgement or the infection rate in the local tick population. The preferred regimen is 100 to 200 mg of doxycycline, twice daily for 20 days. Other treatment options may be appropriate on an individualized basis.
- During the initial visit, clinicians should educate patients regarding the prevention of future tick bites, the potential manifestations of both early and late Lyme disease, and the manifestations of the other tick-borne diseases that they may have contracted because of the recent bite. Patients receiving antibiotic prophylaxis should also be given information describing the symptoms and signs of a *Clostridium difficile* infection and the preventative effect of probiotics. Patients should be encouraged to immediately report the occurrence of all tick-borne disease manifestations and manifestations suggestive of a *C. difficile* infection.

Today, patients expect to be informed of their treatment options. Thus, the review in the *Journal of Emergency Medicine*[230] by Applegren and colleagues would have been stronger had the authors disclosed the ILADS conclusions based on the same evidence.

NEW COMBINATIONS OF ANTIBIOTICS EFFECTIVE IN CULTURE

Because Lyme disease can be difficult to treat, researchers have tested unusual combinations in the laboratory to search for more effective therapies. The goal of these experiments is to figure out why current drugs don't completely eradicate Lyme bacteria. "One possibility is that persisting organisms are not killed by current Lyme antibiotics," according to Feng and colleagues from the Department of Molecular Microbiology and Immunology, Johns Hopkins University.

The authors describe several novel combinations of antibiotics from a Food and Drug Administration drug library, and a National Cancer Institute compound library, that were effective in culture.[231]

- Sulfa drugs combined with other antibiotics were more active than their respective single drugs;
- Sulfa drugs dapsone, sulfachlorpyridazine, and trimethoprim showed very similar activity against stationary phase *Borrelia burgdorferi* enriched in persisters; however, sulfamethoxazole was the least-active drug among the three sulfa drugs tested.

- Four-drug combinations were more active than three-drug combinations.
- Four-drug combinations (dapsone plus minocycline plus cefuroxime plus azithromycin and dapsone plus minocycline plus cefuroxime plus rifampin) showed the best activity.
- Four-sulfa-drug-containing combinations still had considerably less activity than daptomycin plus cefuroxime plus doxycycline used as a positive control, which completely eradicated *B. burgdorferi* stationary phase cells.

Dapsone, trimethoprim, and sulfamethoxazole are on the market for other indications. Dapsone is an antibiotic commonly used in combination with rifampicin and clofazimine for the treatment of leprosy that can lead to hemolysis, methemoglobinemiam, hepatitis, cholestatic jaundice, and rashes. The combination of trimethoprim and sulfamethoxazole are marketed under the names Bactrim and Septra. Sulfachlorpyridazine is not currently used.

Daptomycin is used in the treatment of systemic and life threatening infections of the skin and skin structure, such as *Staphylococcus aureus bacteraemia*, and right-sided *Staphylococcus aureus* endocarditis. It is marketed in the United States under the trade name Cubicin. Side effects include high and low blood pressure, swelling, insomnia, diarrhea, abdominal pain, eosinophilia, dyspnea, injection site reactions, fever, and hypersensitivity. Rare cases of eosinophilic pneumonia have been reported. Myopathy and rhabdomyolysis have occurred in patients concurrently taking statins.

Feng and colleagues stress the need for further study of novel drug combinations both in vitro and in animal models. Eventually such research should lead to better treatment options for physicians and patients.

CASE STUDY: REVERSIBLE COMPLETE HEART BLOCK CAUSED BY LYME DISEASE IN CANADA

*C*omplete heart block, while an uncommon occurrence, is a notable cause of morbidity in the United States. The usual underlying causes of this coronary event include congenital problems or heart disease. But more cases of heart block seem to be occurring due to tick infections.

Take Canada, for example, cases of Lyme disease continue to climb, in part because of the spread of the *Ixodes scapularis* tick by birds.[37] So, it is not surprising to learn Canadian doctors reported their first case of reversible heart block due to Lyme disease in a March 2017 article published in the *American Journal of Medicine*.[232]

"A previously healthy Caucasian 22-year-old male presented to a southern Quebec community hospital with syncopal episodes for one week," according to De l'Étoile-Morel and colleagues from the Department of Internal Medicine, McGill University Health Centre. "He was found to be hypotensive and bradycardic (heart rate 36 beats per minute), due to third degree atrio-ventricular (AV) block, which did not respond to atropine." His cardiac echo was unremarkable.

The young man also presented with multiple, diffusely distributed erythematous patches with central clearing, consistent with early disseminated Lyme disease. His screening test was positive for a Lyme disease serology, but negative by blood smear for Babesia and *Anaplasma* spp.

The man had not traveled outside the province of Quebec. He did, however, have extensive exposure to deeply wooded areas and was in close contact with deer and other wildlife.

"After 48 hours of observation, he underwent a temporary VVI (ventricular pacing and sensing mode) pacemaker insertion," according to l'Étoile-Morel and colleagues. The AV block converted to first degree block after two days of intravenous ceftriaxone treatment. The AV block resolved by day 11, and the pacemaker was removed. He completed a 21-day course of therapy with oral doxycycline. His follow-up Western blot test was positive.

It would have been reasonable to recommend follow-up of this patient to assess for complications of Lyme disease, such as chronic neurologic Lyme disease,[16] Lyme encephalopathy,[17,68] and post treatment Lyme disease syndrome.[130,131]

CASE STUDY: TEMPORARY PACEMAKER EFFECTIVE IN 30-YEAR-OLD WITH HEART BLOCK

A 30-year-old man presented with a syncopal episode with no prodrome (a fainting without warning), shortness of breath, and weakness, according to a July 2017 case study titled "Electrocardiographic Progression of Acute Lyme Disease."

Three weeks earlier, the man had an "insect bite" followed a week later by "chills, sweats, myalgia, back pain, headache, and fatigue," according to Fuster and colleagues from Kingston General Hospital, Queen's University, in Ontario, Canada.[233]

Lyme carditis was diagnosed based on the patient's history, a pulse rate of 38, a high degree of atrial ventricular block, and the absence of ischemia. A temporary transvenous pacemaker was placed through the jugular vein, and the man was admitted to the cardiac unit for monitoring and treatment. Intravenous ceftriaxone was prescribed.[233] The temporary pacemaker was removed on day 6. By day fourteen, the EKG had returned to normal sinus rhythm. The man was discharged and instructed to complete four weeks of antibiotics.

Had the patient gone to a different hospital, the treatment, noted the researchers, might have been quite different. "Quite frequently, these young patients are implanted with permanent pacemakers, given lack of knowledge on the transient nature of the cardiac conduction system inflammation," according to the researchers.[233]

"Most patients presenting with Lyme carditis and new onset arrhythmia do not remember when they have been bitten or they do not have a clear history of tick bite, therefore it is a reasonable decision to investigate those patients for suspicious Lyme disease, especially in high-risk areas or in patients with pathognomonic (characteristic) symptoms like erythema migrans (characteristic migrating rash)," they write.

STEROID USE HAS BEEN ASSOCIATED WITH TREATMENT FAILURE

Several studies have documented the consequences that steroids pose to patients with Lyme disease. Researchers from Massachusetts Eye and Ear and Harvard Medical School published a retrospective study in 2016 that describes "an association between corticosteroid use in acute LDFP [Lyme disease-associated facial palsy] and worse long-term facial function outcomes."[234]

Two-thirds of the 51 study participants had been prescribed steroids, even those with Lyme-associated palsy. "Because corticosteroids are the standard of care for acute viral facial paralysis, it is not surprising that they were prescribed to nearly all patients who were initially misdiagnosed,"[234] the authors explain.

Other studies describe long-term treatment failures following use of steroids.[235,236]

- Three of five late Lyme disease patients treated with corticosteroids were unresponsive to ceftriaxone.[235]
- Three of 24 recurrent Lyme disease patients who failed their initial treatment had been prescribed corticosteroids.[148]
- Treatment failed for Lyme arthritic patients who were

prescribed intramuscular benzathine penicillin following steroids.[236]

So what can physicians learn from this information? "Corticosteroid therapy may simply be a marker for patients with more severe arthritis," because responders generally had lower presedimentation rates and joint-fluid white cell counts," according to Steere and colleagues from the Yale School of Medicine. They add that suppressing the immune system also may have diminished the effective killing of spirochetes.

"Patients unresponsive to ceftriaxone were more likely to have received corticosteroid treatment," according to Dattwyler and colleagues from Stony Brook Medical Center. They conclude that the "association of steroid use with an increased failure rate or worsening of disease is understandable in view of the well-known effects of these agents on the inflammatory and immune responses."[235]

Dattwyler and colleagues advise against the use of steroids in Lyme disease patients. "In view of the strong association between the use of steroids and the lack of response to antibiotic therapy, we believe that glucocorticoids should not be used in the treatment of Lyme borreliosis."[235]

Complications were also reported in a study of dogs infected with *Borrelia burgdorferi*.[237] Dogs succumbed to arthritis after prednisone use, Straubinger and colleagues found. "Corticosteroids inhibit the regulation of cytokines at the DNA level, thus handicapping leukocyte communication during treatment."[238]

PERSISTENCE OF INFECTION MAY DRIVE LYME DISEASE

Several potential causes of elevated chemokines have been identified in Lyme disease patients with persistent symptoms:

- persistence of spirochetal antigens leading to immune dysregulation in CD4+ T-cell subsets
- an autoimmune component based on the findings of antineural antibodies in one cohort of patients with post-treatment Lyme disease syndrome (PTLDS)
- persistence of bacteria[130]

"Studies using rodent and primate models have suggested that the persistence of bacteria and/or spirochetal antigens after antibiotic therapy may drive disease,"[130] according to Aucott from the Division of Rheumatology, Department of Medicine, Johns Hopkins University School of Medicine and the lead author of the study.

Three potential interventions for an elevated chemokine CCL19 were identified:

- medications to treat depression to decrease cytokine levels,
- behavioral interventions for pain and fatigue management,
- cognitive rehabilitation. [130]

The authors point out that a growing number of physicians are retreating their Lyme disease patients with additional antibiotics. These researchers observe, "The use of short-term antibiotic retreatment in the early, post-treatment phase of Lyme disease has yet to be formally tested, although it may be widely applied in clinical practice."[130]

In fact, eight of 107 patients enrolled with confirmed Lyme disease as of 2017 were retreated in the Hopkins study. Two of six Lyme disease patients with PTLDS were retreated (one had a new objective finding and one had a nonfading erythema migrans rash). Six of the 101 Lyme disease patients without PTLDS were retreated. Four of them developed objective findings and two had nonfading erythema migrans rash or new disseminated rash.[123]

SHORT COURSES OF ANTIBIOTICS MAY FAIL TO ERADICATE THE SPIROCHETE

As early as 1990, Logigian and colleagues hypothesized that a two-week course of intravenous ceftriaxone would not successfully eradicate the Lyme bacterium. "The likely reason for relapse is failure to eradicate the spirochete completely with a two-week course of intravenous ceftriaxone therapy,"[16] according to Logigian and colleagues from the Department of Neurology, Tufts University School of Medicine, Boston, Mass.

And, short courses of antibiotics for Lyme disease have failed in other trials.

Other authors, reporting on a 2016 trial in Slovenia, also identified several problems with the two-week course of antibiotics [239]

- Antibiotic therapy was repeated within three to six months "in 20 of 77 patients (26 percent) because of unsatisfactory clinical response to the first treatment (three patients), persistence of CSF cell count $>10\times10^6$ cells/L (eight patients), or both (nine patients)."[239]
- Unfavorable long-term clinical outcomes were observed in nine of 74 patients (12 percent), consisting of

intense/annoying nonspecific symptoms, persistent PFP, or remaining pareses that influenced functioning.[239]

In a 2016 trial in the Netherlands, patients' quality of life was only slightly better following a two-week course of intravenous ceftriaxone. Their quality of life score of 34.8 (out of 50) remained below that of cancer and heart-attack patients and well below the normal of 50 for the general population.

More than a third of early Lyme disease patients treated with a three-week course of antibiotics remained ill at a six-month follow-up in a 2013 trial at Johns Hopkins. At six months, 36 percent of 66 patients reported new-onset fatigue, 20 percent widespread pain, and 45 percent neurocognitive difficulties.[19]

These studies suggest physicians should consider using more effective treatments than the short courses of antibiotics described in the Slovenian, Netherlands, and U.S. trials, in order to avoid treatment failure.[19,125,239]

DIVERSITY OF STRAINS MAY EXPLAIN TREATMENT FAILURES

*I*n previous essays, readers have learned of three potential reasons why treatments for Lyme may fail. Those reasons include: delayed treatment,[148,240,241] exposure to steroids,[148,235] and the presence of co-infections [60] can potentially explain why some patients fail to get better with treatment. Now comes another potential cause for failed treatment: Strain virulence.[48,242-248]

Differing genotypes of *Borrelia burgdorferi* may play a role in strain virulence.[245] For example, three different Outer Surface Protein C (OspC) have been identified on the surface of the spirochete; and each OspC exhibits a different virulence.[244]

Seinost and colleagues at the Department of Medicine, State University of New York at Stony Brook noted those OspC differences in a 1999 paper titled "Four clones of Borrelia burgdorferi sensu stricto cause invasive infection in humans,"[244]

The genetic diversity of *B. burgdorferi* may be getting worse, as well. "The Lyme disease bacteria is evolving in response to the immune defense of its natural hosts (including rodents and birds)," says Walter.[249] An expanding genetic diversity adds to concerns over strain virulence. "Complex interactions between co-infecting strains and the host may result in mixed infections with a range of virulence outcomes."

This all calls to mind an observation made by the American paleontologist Stephen Jay Gould. "The most outstanding feature of life's history is that through 3.5 billion years this has remained, really, a bacterial planet."[250]

NEW DRUG APPROACHES IDENTIFIED TO COMBAT LYME PERSISTER CELLS

In 2015 and 2016, researchers from Johns Hopkins University published findings from *in vitro* studies which suggest novel treatment approaches, including multiple drug combinations, may be effective in treating lingering symptoms of Lyme disease.[251,252]

Feng and colleagues from Hopkins hypothesized that when *Borrelia burgdorferi* is confronted with certain stressors, such as starvation or exposure to antibiotics, the spirochete can transform into a "round body" or "persister" form.[252] "These round bodies appear to have both lower metabolism and greater resistance to antibiotic treatment," according to the authors. When examined *in vitro*, the forms appear to be resistant to customary first-line antibiotics used to treat Lyme disease, hence their ability to persist in the body.

The authors identify novel drug combinations they believe are effective in combating round body persisters in vitro. "We identified 23 drug candidates that have higher activity against the round bodies of *B. burgdorferi* than either amoxicillin or doxycycline," report Feng and colleagues.[252] "It is most likely that a single drug may not effectively kill all bacterial populations including morphological variants."

Combination treatment that included daptomycin was found to be the most effective in these *in vitro* studies. "Daptomycin plus doxycycline and cefoperazone eradicated the most resistant microcolony form of B. burgdorferi persisters, and did not yield viable spirochetes upon subculturing, suggesting durable killing that was not achieved by any other two or three drug combinations."[253]

Their model also found artemisinin, ciprofloxacin, nifuroxime, fosfomycin, chlortetracycline, sulfacetamide, sulfamethoxypyridazine, and sulfathiozole to be effective.[252]

It remains unclear how important round body forms are *in vivo*. Feng and colleagues note that round bodies have been described in human infections, including brain tissue,[254] but their significance remains unclear.[255] "Some have suggested that these round body forms might be a protective mechanism to overcome adverse environmental conditions." the researchers wrote.

It's also unclear which, if any, antibiotics or combinations would be effective until further *in vitro* and *in vivo* research is done. Several of the drugs have not been approved for human use.

• *Daptomycin* is an intravenous antibiotic used in the treatment of systemic and life-threatening infections caused by Gram-positive organisms.

• *Clofazimine* is used in combination with rifampicin and dapsone as a multi-drug therapy for the treatment of leprosy. It is no longer commercially available in the United States.

• *Nifuroxime* is a topical nitrofuran with antifungal properties available in some countries worldwide.

• *Fosfomycin* (marketed in the United States under the brand name Monurol) is a synthetic, broad-spectrum, bactericidal antibiotic for oral administration indicated only for the treatment of uncomplicated urinary tract infections in women due to susceptible strains of *Escherichia coli* and *Enterococcus faecalis*.

• *Chlortetracycline* is a tetracycline antibiotic for use in beef cattle, non-lactating dairy cattle, and sheep.

• *Sulfacetamide* is a 10-percent topical lotion approved for the treatment of acne and seborrheic dermatitis.

• *Sulfamethoxypyridazine* is a sulfonamide antibacterial prescribed for vaginal irritation and severe acute thrush.

• *Sulfathiazole* is a short-acting sulfa drug used until less toxic alternatives were discovered. It is still occasionally used, sometimes in aquariums.

These in vitro studies have introduced new approaches worthy of further study. Unfortunately, developing novel treatment regimens for Lyme disease takes much time and effort; and that effort is often a costly endeavor.

ANTIBIOTICS OR LIFE-LONG IMMUNOSUPPRESSIVE THERAPY?

*D*octors at Massachusetts General Hospital, Boston, reviewed the records of patients referred to its Rheumatology clinic, and noted 30 patients who developed systemic autoimmune joint disease following Lyme disease. "All 30 patients had been treated with antibiotic regimens for Lyme disease, as recommended by the Infectious Diseases Society of America (IDSA)," Arvikar and colleagues pointed out. "Generally, this consisted of a 21-day course of oral doxycycline for early Lyme disease," they wrote. "And 13 of the 24 patients (54 percent) with early Lyme disease received additional courses of oral antibiotic therapy, with a maximum of four months of treatment."[256]

The authors assumed that the persistent *Borrelia burgdorferi* infection had been eradicated. "Fifteen had rheumatoid arthritis (RA), 13 had psoriatic arthritis (PsA), and two had peripheral spondyloarthropathy (SpA)," the researchers noted.[256]

Instead of additional antibiotics, the patients were prescribed anti-inflammatory therapies, primarily disease-modifying anti-rheumatic drugs (DMARDs) to slow down disease progression. "These treatments included steroids (3 percent), NSAIDS (20 percent),

DMARDs (57 percent), most commonly methotrexate, but also TNF-inhibitors, or combinations of these agents," report the authors.[256]

They authors granted that their cases could be a coincidence, "The occurrence of RA, PsA, or SpA following soon after Lyme disease may simply be a coincidence, as these autoimmune disorders are relatively common and Lyme disease is epidemic in our geographic area. Massachusetts General Hospital is located in the northeastern United States, an area endemic for tick-borne illnesses.

The doctors advised immunosuppressive therapy based on the belief that "there is increasing evidence that earlier aggressive treatment of inflammatory arthritis is associated with improved radiographic outcomes and chances of sustained remission." Remission typically is defined as disappearance of signs and symptoms.

However, immunosuppressive therapy raises concerns for patients who develop systemic autoimmune joint disease following Lyme disease. Long-term follow-up information is sparse for these patients. Only four of their 30 subjects with systemic autoimmune joint disease following Lyme disease developed drug-free remission.

While the authors reported that patients with arthritis as an outcome had "well-controlled" arthritis, they don't define what that means.

Finally, the authors concluded that "none of the patients had reactivation of infection." However, they don't offer a well-defined criterion to assure other doctors that their patients with systemic autoimmune joint disease don't indeed suffer from a persistent infection.

The authors describe the case of one patient to highlight the difficulties of determining whether to treat with immunosuppressive medications or antibiotics. The patient developed Rheumatoid Factor (RF) and ACPA positive rheumatoid arthritis initially, and had complete remission of rheumatoid arthritis with methotrexate treatment. But the patient stopped this medication and sought further treatment for Lyme disease elsewhere with prolonged courses of multiple antibiotics. Three years later, the patient returned in a wheelchair and had developed radiographically evident erosions, as well as deformities and contractures in multiple joints.

"Given a choice between [Lyme arthritis] and a chronic illness that may require lifelong immunosuppressive therapy, it is not surprising that patients would find [Lyme arthritis] a more attractive diagnosis," say Arvikar and colleagues "Delaying appropriate DMARD treatment of autoimmune joint disorders by pursuing further therapy with antibiotic agents may lead to poorer clinical outcomes."

The other 29 patients described by the authors leave open this question: Could delaying appropriate antibiotic therapy, by pursuing immunosuppressive therapy, have led to poorer clinical outcomes?

PROBIOTICS MAY HELP WARD OFF CLOSTRIDIUM DIFFICILE DIARRHEA

Clostridium difficile is a leading cause of hospital- and community-acquired associated diarrhea. *C. difficile* is a toxin-producing anaerobic rod bacterium that has been associated with severe presentations, including "toxic megacolon, leukemoid reaction, severe hypoalbuminemia, septic shock, and death," according to Lau, lead author of a 2016 study published in the *International Journal of General Medicine*.[257] This is an important study for patients with Lyme disease who routinely need long-term antibiotic therapy.

This recent study demonstrated the effectiveness of probiotics in warding off *C. difficile*-associated diarrhea in children and adults. Each of the probiotics examined in the meta-analysis was beneficial. "Lactobacillus, Saccharomyces, and a mixture of probiotics were all beneficial in reducing the risk of developing *C. difficile*-associated diarrhea (63.7 percent, 58.5 percent, and 58.2 percent reduction, respectively)."

The authors conclude that "probiotic supplementation is associated with a significant reduction in the risk of developing *C. difficile*-associated diarrhea in patients receiving antibiotics." However, more studies are needed to determine the optimal dosage and strain of probiotics.[257]

Probiotics have also been shown to play a therapeutic role in common disorders for diarrhea due to irritable bowel syndrome and ulcerative colitis.[257]

"Commensal bacteria inhibit enteric pathogens and may help suppress the growth and invasion of pathogenic bacteria, thereby improving intestinal barrier function. Probiotics also modulate proinflammatory cytokines, which help regulate immune responses and maintain homeostasis,"[257] wrote Lau and colleagues.

Doctors have had to weigh the risk of acquiring *C. difficile*-associated diarrhea from antibiotics against the risk of a persistent tick-borne infection. Antibiotic therapy for Lyme disease has led to *C. difficile*-associated diarrhea.[258-260] And, one death associated with *C. difficile* in a Lyme disease patient has been reported.[259]

Some doctors have determined that the risk of a persistent infection[76,77,130] for 300,000 patients in the United States each year outweighs the risk of *C. difficile*-associated diarrhea.[69]

Effective treatments for *C. difficile*-associated diarrhea are available if probiotics are not successful, such as oral metronidazole and oral vancomycin. Fecal microbiota transplantation has been described, as well. In fact, Lau and colleagues cite a study where fecal transplantation was more effective than vancomycin (90 percent vs. 26 percent, $P<0.0001$).[261]

CASE STUDY: ANXIOUS WITH SUICIDAL THOUGHTS AND A HISTORY OF LYME DISEASE

One of the most challenging aspects in treating Lyme disease patients lies in the ability to decipher whether a patient's current health complaints could be attributed to Lyme infection. This challenge becomes even greater when a person has coexisting psychiatric symptoms.

In a 2015 article titled "New-Onset Panic, Depression with Suicidal Thoughts and Somatic Symptoms in a Patient with a History of Lyme Disease," researchers highlight the complexity of evaluating and treating a patient with a history of suspected Lyme disease who presented with neuropsychiatric symptoms.[262]

Garakani and colleagues present the case of a 37-year-old employed man who was admitted to an emergency department with new-onset panic, depression with suicidal thoughts, and somatic symptoms including a three-month history of palpitations, tremulousness, chest pressure, choking sensation, and an intense fear of dying.[262]

The patient also reported back pain and muscle spasms, weakness and tingling in his arms and legs, general fatigue, poor sleep, low energy, loss of interest in his job and social activities, loss of appetite, and a

10-pound weight loss. He had remained ill despite being treated with antidepressants and anti-anxiety medications for the previous two months.

He reported a history of Lyme disease two years prior when he developed fatigue, tinnitus, headaches, fever, and other flu-like symptoms a month after removing a tick from his leg. The patient had a positive Lyme ELISA antibody. His symptoms were said to have resolved after a three-week course of doxycycline, 100 mg twice daily. However, he continued to suffer from anxiety and neuromuscular pains and visited the emergency department several more times.

The patient was eventually admitted to inpatient psychiatry for depression and suicidal ideas, and he was prescribed antidepressants, anti-anxiety medications, and a beta-blocker. Nevertheless, he continued to complain of cramping, flank pain, fatigue, arthritic knee pain, anxiety, poor attention and focus, and panic.

Garakani and colleagues report, "He was very forgetful at home and would often not recall having taken his medications or where he had left common household items," and he was "frustrated by the persistence of his neurological symptoms, which further contributed to his hopelessness and passive thoughts of dying."

On day 8, after his mood had improved, the patient was discharged. At that time, the man still complained of fatigue, weakness, back and leg spasms, "shooting pains" in his hands, and pain and tingling "rising up" in his body, according to the authors.[262]

Despite having visited multiple internists and neurologists, the man continued to have cognitive deficits upon discharge. Evaluations included negative Lyme disease Western blot tests.

The patient continued to seek treatment with other specialists and was diagnosed with Lyme disease. He was tested at IGeneX Laboratories in California. Results indicated he was positive for *Borrelia* on Bands 31 and 34 and babesiosis. These bands have not been included in the CDC seroepidemiologic criteria. There is no record of whether the treating physician used clinical judgment or laboratory testing in making the diagnosis.

After a six-month course of oral antibiotics, including three months of tetracycline and three months of azithromycin and fluconazole, the man's cognitive deficits improved. He no longer reported having panic attacks, periods of hopelessness, or suicidal thoughts, and he could stop his psychiatric medications.

The authors focused on a cognitive behavioral approach. The patient still felt "despondent and frustrated by the lack of improvement in his physical symptoms." He had been forced to leave his job and go on disability, and he continued to have fatigue, weakness, low energy, pain and spasms in his back and upper legs, and nonspecific joint pain, state Garakani and colleagues.[262]

The authors did not discuss the option of treating babesiosis, despite his history of a positive Babesia test. A combination of azithromycin and atovaquone has been effective in treating patients coinfected with Lyme disease and babesiosis.[60]

The authors also did not discuss the option of treating with intravenous antibiotics, despite reports that spirochete can cross the blood-brain barrier. Intravenous ceftriaxone has been effective in treating chronic neurologic Lyme disease and Lyme encephalopathy.

This case study offers insight into the complexity of evaluating and treating a patient with neuropsychiatric symptoms and a history of Lyme disease. Although the evaluation and treatment may have been well thought out, additional treatment options could have been discussed with the patient.

Alternatively, the 37-year-old man might have benefited from a combination of cognitive behavioral therapy and antibiotics.

LONG DIAGNOSTIC DELAYS THWART SUCCESS RATE OF LYME TREATMENT

*T*he old adage: *Once bitten, twice shy* takes on a new meaning in an era of tick infections, because once bitten by a tick, people find doctors shy away from diagnosing and treating Lyme disease. In fact, in a 2008 article, Fallon and colleagues reported diagnostic delays were averaging two years in patients who were later diagnosed with Lyme encephalopathy.[17]

Those Lyme encephalopathy patients, Fallon's group discovered remained ill an average of nine years after onset of the disease, with a poor quality of life on an SF-36 measure.[17]

Just a year earlier, in 2007, Cameron reported diagnostic delays averaging 1.8 years in patients who had failed treatment for Lyme disease. Each of the patients in his case-control study was serologically confirmed with five out of 10 positive IgG western blot bands.[148]

The patients in the Cameron study who failed treatment included:

- a 34-year-old man with an erythema migrans rash who was

tested one week after the rash appeared but had been ill for eight years
- a 16-year-old girl with Epstein-Barr and strep infections who had been ill for eight years
- a 57-year-old man with a tick bite followed by a swollen right knee, which was presumed to be a meniscus tear, who had been ill for six years
- a 16-year-old boy who presented with Bell's palsy and complained of performing poorly in school, who had been ill for six years
- a 35-year-old man who exhibited symptoms consistent with Lyme disease but was told by two clinicians that he did not have Lyme and remained ill for three years
- a 42-year-old woman whose spinal tap results were negative and had been ill for three years[148]

Lyme disease patients in the Cameron case-control series required more extensive treatment.[148]

These studies show physicians who shy away from treating symptoms of Lyme disease leave their patients to suffer while they further seek a correct diagnosis and treatment. And delaying a diagnosis also means patients become sicker, and therefore need more intense treatment options.

HUNDREDS OF DOCTORS PRESCRIBING LONGER COURSES OF THERAPY

A handful of hot-button issues surrounding Lyme disease continue to ignite debates within the medical community. Among them is the duration of time required to effectively treat the disease.

The Infectious Diseases Society of America (IDSA) has long insisted that a maximum antibiotic course of 21 days is sufficient to eradicate the Lyme bacterium, while the International Lyme and Associated Diseases Society (ILADS) recommends a longer course of antibiotics with duration dependent on a patient's response to therapy.[70]

So, what treatment approach are physicians adopting in their clinical practices? A study by Tseng and colleagues, published in the August 2015 issue of *Clinical Infectious Diseases*, aimed to answer that question. They discovered, after reviewing insurance claims data, "that the use of extended courses of antibiotics and multiple antibiotics in the treatment of Lyme disease has increased in recent years."[220]

The study examined the incidence and patterns of prolonged antibiotic treatment in Lyme disease patients in the northeastern

United States during the years 2004-2006 and 2010-2012. The authors retrospectively analyzed health-insurance claims for patients receiving Lyme disease treatment in 14 high-prevalence states including: Connecticut, Delaware, Maine, Maryland, Massachusetts, Minnesota, New Hampshire, New Jersey, New York, Pennsylvania, Rhode Island, Vermont, Virginia, and Wisconsin.[220]

Since the study was all-inclusive and not restricted by patients testing positive on the two-tier test, it offered unique insight into actual treatment practices and was more representative of the patient population afflicted with Lyme disease.

Eighteen percent of Lyme disease patients were treated for more than five weeks. The actual length of time patients were prescribed antibiotics was an average of 86 days. Treatment duration ranged from 35-to-404 days.[220]

Nearly half of Lyme disease patients treated with extended therapy (48.8 percent) were treated with more than two antibiotics. Doxycycline was prescribed for as many as 74.4 percent of patients. Azithromycin was prescribed for 11.5 percent of patients. Amoxicillin and cefuroxime were also prescribed. The study did not look at additional antibiotics, such as minocycline and tetracycline, typically prescribed to treat other tick-borne illnesses.[220]

The study also found that 43 percent of patients were switched from one antibiotic to another, while 18 percent were prescribed combinations of antibiotics.[220]

It was not a surprise that the study identified doctors who prescribed extended therapy for a significant number of Lyme disease patients. Those 16 doctors (three percent) treated more than 20 percent of the Lyme disease patients who were prescribed extended antibiotic treatment.[220]

It was a surprise to find that hundreds of other providers in the northeastern United States, identified in a single insurance database, also prescribed extended antibiotics. In all, 472 doctors treated the remaining 80 percent of Lyme disease patients with extended therapy.

Also surprising, the prescribing patterns did not differ between the 16 doctors, who treated more than 20 percent of the Lyme disease patients, and their 472 colleagues when assessing the average number of antibiotic exposure days, the number of refills in the longest drug era, and the combination of antibiotics prescribed.

The authors did not address why 488 doctors treated their Lyme disease patients longer than the 21 days recommended by the 2006 IDSA evidence-based guidelines.[70]

Medical societies continue to debate the optimal treatment regimen. In the meantime, hundreds of doctors are choosing extended antibiotic therapy for select patients.

COULD MONOCLONAL ANTIBODIES PREVENT LYME DISEASE?

Researchers say they've had promising results in developing a method to prevent people from becoming infected with *Borrelia burgdorferi*, the cause of Lyme disease. It doesn't involve a vaccine, but rather a process that stimulates the immune system to ward off infections.

Klempner and colleagues at MassBiologics, the University of Massachusetts' nonprofit vaccine-development arm, describe a study where lab-developed monoclonal antibodies prevented Lyme disease in mice.

Klempner's group first discussed its findings with reporter Maggie Fox of *NBC News*,[225] while they were in San Diego, California on Oct. 9, 2015, attending a conference with infectious disease experts.[225]

One year later, MassBiologics had refined the protocol and named it Lyme PReP. In a June 2016 newsletter titled, *What a Year!* and published by the Massachusetts Society for Medical Research (MSMR), readers learned the difference between a vaccine and Klempner's goal of designing a monoclonal antibody protocol.[263]

"The basic purpose of a vaccine is to protect the body against a specific infection. Vaccines achieve this goal by introducing a weakened form of the bacteria or virus to the immune system. This allows the immune system to recognize particular proteins characteristic of the disease and create specialized proteins, known as antibodies, which will fight the infection." [263]

But Klempner wants to develop a different approach, the newsletter explained. "Since they are aiming at protecting people from getting Lyme disease they have called their approach pre-exposure prophylaxis, or PREP for short. Unlike a vaccine which stimulates the production of a large cast of antibodies, PREP introduces only the specific antibody needed for protection. It is a more difficult approach because it requires researchers to first identify a single antibody to prevent infection."[263]

Klempner found the mouse study encouraging. He told NBC News his company was laying the groundwork to start testing its monoclonal antibody protocol in people in 2016. [225] Yet in the 2016 newsletter, Klempner were still refining their antibody protocol. Klempner noted "This process usually takes a decade," says Dr. Klempner. "We are well on our way." Dr. Klempner hopes the antibody for Lyme PrEP will be available to the general public in about 3 to 5 years. That would mean somewhere between 2019 and 2021.[225]

Hopefully investigators at MassBiologics will address several outstanding questions:[264]

- Will the monoclonal antibodies work for the growing number of different strains of the *B. burgdorferi* infection?
- Will the monoclonal antibodies work for new species, such as *Borrelia miyamotoi*, which is related to the bacteria causing tick-borne relapsing fever described by the Centers for Disease Control and Prevention?[265]
- Will monoclonal antibodies be developed for other tick-borne illnesses, such as babesiosis and anaplasmosis?

- Will people exhibit any side effects not evident in the mice?
- Will the monoclonal antibodies be affordable? The NBC News report points out that they often cost upward of $100,000 a year. But Klempner said the university's goal is to make the treatment available cheaply.

CASE STUDY: 67-YEAR-OLD MAN AVOIDS SURGERY FOR ARTHRITIS

*E*arly and prompt diagnosis, and adequate antibiotic treatment, allowed doctors to avoid taking additional and aggressive surgical intervention for a patient with a partial knee replacement. That patient later presented with complications caused by Lyme disease. The case was reported in 2016 by Wright and colleagues from the Division of Infectious Disease, Department of Medicine, Memorial Medical Center, York, Pennsylvania, in *The Journal of Arthroplasty*. The case highlights the need "to further investigate and interpret unexpected findings in clinical practice,"[266] the authors wrote.

The physicians describe a 67-year-old avid outdoorsman from central Pennsylvania with a three-month history of progressive left knee pain and swelling.[266] Ten months earlier, the patient had undergone surgery for unicompartmental joint arthroplasty (partial knee replacement) of his left knee to correct the problem caused by advanced single compartment degenerative arthritis.

He presented with a moderate joint effusion (known in lay terms as water on the knee). Aspiration of the knee revealed a turbid purulent pleocytosis (cloudy, pussy fluid filled with white blood cells) with 91.8 percent neutrophils (a type of white blood cell) and a positive Borrelia burgdorferi polymerase chain reaction (PCR). Serologic tests were positive for B. burgdorferi by antibody enzyme immunoassay screen, and 10 of 10 IgG western blot bands, according to Wright and colleagues.[266]

The authors summarize their concern over the seriousness of an infection. "Periprosthetic joint infection is a devastating complication following joint arthroplasty that causes significant morbidity." Estimated cumulative incidence is 1 to 2 percent for hips and knees.[266]

Doctors elected to treat the 67-year-old man with antibiotics rather than surgical incision and drainage or excision arthroplasty. They initiated 100 mg of oral doxycycline twice daily until testing confirmed the Lyme diagnosis. The treatment was converted to a six-week course of 2 grams intravenous ceftriaxone daily.[266]

The antibiotic treatment was successful. "Clinically, the patient had cessation of his knee pain, resolution of joint effusion, normalization of synovial infection and inflammatory parameters, and negative end-of-therapy detection of *B. burgdorferi* DNA by PCR," according to Wright and colleagues.[266]

The authors say it's unclear whether those results could be achieved with any of the oral antimicrobial agents recommended by the Infectious Diseases Society of America (IDSA).[266]

They caution that their strategy of prolonged intravenous antibiotics might not be effective in other types of joint arthroplasties. "Although this patient's clinical outcome was achieved without the need for surgical incision and drainage or staged excision arthroplasty procedure, it is unclear whether this same strategy would produce similar results in patients with other types of joint arthroplasties."

More than 82,660 patients underwent total knee arthroplasty across the Medicare and United Health Care populations from 2009 to 2011, at a cost exceeding $10 billion a year.[267] This case begs the question: Could other arthroplasties be caused by underlying Lyme infections and prevented by antibiotic therapy?

AZITHROMYCIN GEL FAILS TO PREVENT LYME DISEASE

Three former employees of Novartis Pharmaceuticals—a chemist, a pharmacist and an economist—created a company called IxodesAG in an effort to develop a topical antibiotic for tick bites.[268]

In 2015, the U.S. Food and Drug Administration "designated the company's lead product candidate, Ixogel®, as a Qualified Infectious Disease Product (QIDP) for the prevention of Lyme Disease after a tick bite."[269] In a press release, the Swiss based company noted: "The QIDP designation will make Ixogel® eligible to benefit from certain incentives as provided under the Generating Antibiotic Incentives Now (GAIN) program. These incentives include FDA priority review and eligibility for fast-track status and—providing that FDA approval is obtained—Ixogel® would be eligible for an additional five-year extension of Hatch-Waxman patent exclusivity."[269]

Yet, a 2016 study conducted in Germany and Austria, funded by IxodesAG, and published in *The Lancet Infectious Diseases*, concluded Ixogel®, did not perform well as a first-response after a tick bite.[270]

Within 72-hours of a known tick bite, researchers applied the 10 percent azithromycin Ixogel® to the bite site for three consecutive days.261 Unfortunately, the topical treatment failed to prevent infection from spreading. The authors noted, "The primary outcome was the number of treatment failures, defined as erythema migrans, seroconversion, or both, in participants who were seronegative at baseline, had no further tick bites during the study."

And while acknowledging the gel "was well tolerated and had a good safety profile," the researchers stopped the trial early "because an improvement in the primary endpoint in the group receiving azithromycin was not reached."

The trial only demonstrated that the gel could prevent or delay a few erythema migrans rashes in a post-hoc analysis of a subset of 134 patients bitten by a tick.[270] The authors were able to prevent six rashes if the gel was applied after a tick bite. The gel delayed the onset of rashes by 33 and 51 days, respectively, in an additional two subjects.[270]

Researchers at IxodesAG continue to refine Ixogel®. The company wants to address what it calls "the perplexing finding" about the *Borrelia* bacteria. It remains "at, or close to, the tick bite for several days," according to the company's site, "hence, being a formidable target for massive pharmaceutical attack through topical delivery of antibiotics."[271]

It would be nice to have a quick fix to prevent Lyme disease following a tick bite. But treatment with azithromycin gel is not the answer. Based on this trial, the gel should not be used to try to prevent Lyme disease.

SECTION X. SPECIAL CONCERNS FOR CHILDREN

*A*uthor Richard Louv, in his book titled *Last Child in the Woods*, writes about the nature deficit of children in this wired world. "Direct exposure to nature is essential for healthy childhood development and for the physical and emotional health of children and adults," wrote Louv.[272] Sadly, in this new world of tick infections, Louv's observations come with a caveat to take precautions even when they are out in your own backyard.

Children make up about a quarter of all Lyme disease cases reported each year. And if kids develop chronic Lyme disease, they potentially face a lifetime of suffering. The following conversations focus on concerns which impact children hardest: difficulties of diagnosis, the need for prompt, aggressive treatment, and the importance of prevention.

Readers will find of particular interest, two case studies highlighting kids with behavioral and psychiatric symptoms resulting from infection, which were initially misdiagnosed as typical challenges of childhood.

CHILDREN AT GREATEST RISK FOR BEING BITTEN BY TICKS

*C*hildren make up an estimated 25 percent of all Lyme disease cases in the United States, according to the Centers for Disease Control and Prevention (CDC).[273] Despite the oft-made recommendation for tick checks, the number of children and adolescents developing Lyme disease continues to rise.

A 2016 study published in *Vector Borne Zoonotic Diseases* confirms that children remain most at risk of being bitten by a tick. Xu and colleagues report children younger than age 9 remain the group most at-risk for being bitten. Both nymphs and adults were identified.

- Nearly 200 ticks were collected from children below age 5.
- Another 200 ticks were collected from children ages 5 to 9.
- Nearly 90 ticks were collected from adolescents.[274]

The most common bites were from deer ticks. Of the 3,551 tick bites, 89 percent were by deer ticks. And, 98 percent of the 1,700 adult ticks submitted were female.

The overall infection rates for *Borrelia burgdorferi, Anaplasmosis phagocytophilum*, and *Babesia microti* in human-biting ticks were 29.6

percent, 4.6 percent, and 1.8 percent, respectively.[274] The investigators did not check for other infections, such as *Bartonella henselae* or *Borrelia miyamotoi*.

The most bites were reported in the spring and fall, when children participate in school activities and sports. The adult tick bites peaked during two periods: April – June, representing questing activity of the overwintering tick population, and October – December, representing large autumnal populations.[275] Between April and October, 360 nymphs were received, with a clear peak in June.

TICK BITES: YOUNG KIDS AND THE ELDERLY HAVE SOMETHING IN IN COMMON

Young children and the elderly are at the greatest risk of Lyme disease in the United States, according to the Centers for Disease Control and Prevention (CDC). That finding is backed up by a study of emergency department (ED) admissions in New Hampshire.[276]

From 2010 to 2014, more than 10,359 tick bite encounters were documented in 25 acute care hospitals in New Hampshire. All but one acute care hospital in the state participated.

Young kids and the elderly were the most likely to have been evaluated in the ED. Of all tick-bite-related ED encounters, 6 percent and 22 percent occurred in children 5 and younger and adults 65 and older, respectively. Those findings were reported by Daly and colleagues from the Bureau of Infectious Disease Control, New Hampshire Department of Health and Human Services, Concord, New Hampshire, in the journal *Zoonoses Public Health*.

Young kids and the elderly are arguably the most difficult to diagnose if they develop an atypical rash or another manifestation of Lyme disease. Older children and adolescents were also commonly diagnosed with Lyme disease in the emergency room.

The authors highlight the need for provider and patient education. "Results of ED data analyses can be used to target education, in particular for ED providers and the public through timely distribution of evidence-based educational materials and training," according to Daly and colleagues.[276]

It would be reasonable to inform patients that a single 200 mg dose of doxycycline can prevent a rash but has not been proven to prevent other manifestations of Lyme disease or co-infections.[195]

ONE IN THREE TICKS REMOVED FROM CHILDREN IS ENGORGED

Since many children, despite the influence of technology, spend time outdoors; even in their backyards; it is not surprising to learn that one study, conducted in Massachusetts by Xu et.al., revealed 35.6 percent of attached ticks were engorged in children younger than 9 years.[275] And, the longer a tick is attached, the greater the chance the spirochetes will multiply in the midgut of the tick and then travel to the salivary glands for transmission. The chances of contracting Lyme disease from an engorged tick are 20 percent in an endemic area.[277]

How long it takes a tick to transmit disease after attaching is still unknown. In 2015, independent British researcher Michael Cook reviewed the literature on tick attachment time and the transmission of Lyme disease. Cook concluded, "The claims that removal of ticks within 24 hours or 48 hours of attachment will effectively prevent LB (*Lyme Borrealis*) are not supported by the published data, and the minimum tick attachment time for transmission of LB in humans has never been established."[278]

What researchers do know is that an engorged tick is female; she has fed on a host, and she has potentially transmitted a disease, or multiple diseases. The Minnesota Department of Health provides easy to understand information about tick biology and feeding. [279]

- The adult female ticks feed and mate on large animals in the fall or early spring. The female lays her eggs, then dies.
- If the ticks did not get a blood meal in the fall, they go dormant over winter and seek a meal in the spring. A frost does not kill blacklegged ticks. Adults may become active as soon as it is above freezing. They are occasionally spotted during a temporary thaw in the winter.
- As female ticks feed over the course of several days, their bodies slowly enlarge with blood (engorge). Adult females infected with disease agents as larvae or nymphs may transmit disease during this feeding.
- Male ticks attach, but do not feed or become engorged. Because the adult males do not take a blood meal, they do not transmit Lyme disease, human anaplasmosis, or babesiosis.

When one in three children have an engorged tick attached; and studies indicate the chance of contracting Lyme disease from an engorged tick increases to 20 percent in an endemic area; [277] then it's a good indicator that preventive measures, such as doing routine tick checks, are not working.

ONLY 12 PERCENT OF CHILDREN REPORT ALWAYS CHECKING FOR TICKS

Researchers from the Division of Rheumatology at the Harvard Medical School wanted to know how often children checked themselves for ticks after playing outdoors. To that end, the Shadick and colleagues selected 3570 "students in grades 2-5 in 19 elementary schools" who lived in a Lyme endemic area to participate in a study.[280]

As designed, "1562 received the intervention, and 2008 were controls." The educational intervention consisted of a "short, in-class educational program" on how to prevent Lyme disease. Researchers wrote, student "knowledge, attitudes, and self-reported preventive behaviors were surveyed before implementing the program and 1 year later.[280]

When asked how often they check themselves for ticks, 56.8 percent of children responded "sometimes," 25.8 percent said "usually," and only 12 percent responded "always." When asked who helps them check for ticks most of the time, 77.8 percent said a grown-up at home, while 14.6 percent said they checked themselves. Only 2 percent said a grown-up at school checked for ticks, while 4.4 percent said they were not checked at all.[280]

The researchers discovered "All children in classes receiving the intervention reported an increase in precautionary behavior, [and a] positive attitude toward taking precautions." Interestingly, they also noted, "Two LD cases were confirmed during the follow-up period, one in the intervention group and one in the control."[280]

The study was published in 2016, in *Vector Borne Zoonotic Diseases*. Its findings clearly demonstrate the need for education to prevent tick bites of children.

A 2015 study conducted by researchers in the Netherlands, and published in a similarly named journal, *Vector-Borne and Zoonotic Diseases,* noted "effective measures to control tick populations or vaccines for LB are not yet available. Therefore, behavioral measures including avoidance of areas inhabited by ticks, performing routine body checks, using protective clothing, and the application of tick repellents are of great importance." Beaujean and colleagues continued, "Unfortunately, acceptance and uptake of many of these preventive behaviors are currently low."[281]

The researchers concluded, "As long as there are no effective measures for controlling tick populations and there is no vaccine available, we rely solely on health education and communication efforts to prevent tick bites and LB (*Lyme Borrealis*). We call on researchers and funders to prioritize research in the field of public health interventions for tick bites and LB because, in the words of Benjamin Franklin, 'an ounce of prevention is worth a pound of cure.'"[281]

CHILDREN HOSPITALIZED WITH LYME DISEASE

When is Lyme disease diagnosed in children not really Lyme disease? That's what authors of a 2016 study titled "False Positive Lyme Disease IgM Immunoblots in Children" which was published in the *Journal of Pediatrics*. The study, conducted by Paul Lantos of Duke University, and two physicians from Boston Children's Hospital, noted that "almost one-third of positive IgM immunoblots" in adults were unlikely to have Lyme disease, so what about children?[282]

To find the answer, researchers looked at seven years of data from Boston Children's Hospital, the researchers "examined the clinical presentations of children from a highly endemic region with a positive IgM immunoblot alone."[282]

Using data from the hospital's electronic data warehouse, the researchers included in their study "individuals 21 years of age and younger who had a Lyme EIA obtained between January 1, 2007, and June 30, 2014. We included multiple Lyme disease tests from the same patient over the study period."[282]

Interestingly, the researchers wrote, the institutional review board at

Boston Children's Hospital "approved the study protocol with waiver of informed consent."268

Lantos and colleagues noted that between Jan. 1, 2007, and June 30, 2014, "7289 Lyme disease tests were obtained from 7043 unique patients. Reflex immunoblots were performed for the 1216 (17%) specimens with a positive or equivocal EIA result. Of the tests with confirmatory immunoblots performed, we identified 167 cases with positive IgM and negative IgG immunoblot result (2.2% of Lyme tests) from 167 unique children."282

Looking more closely at the 167 patients the researchers identified, they collected the following date:

- 58 (35%) had EM,
- 71 (43%) had signs compatible with early-disseminated Lyme disease,
- 14 (8%) with late Lyme disease
- 24 (14%) had nonspecific clinical presentations.

Furthermore, "Of the 71 children with signs compatible with early-disseminated Lyme disease, 38 had radiculoneuropathy, 28 had meningitis, and 5 had carditis." Researchers then concluded, "The 10 children who had signs lasting more than 60 days did not have Lyme disease. Additionally, the 14 children with arthritis and the 24 with nonspecific signs of ≤60 days duration did not have Lyme disease. Only 3 children had a repeat immunoblot performed at the study institution, of which 1 result was negative, and 2 had a persistently positive IgM and negative IgG result. Overall, 119 of the 167 children with a positive IgM immunoblot alone had Lyme disease (71.2%; 95% CI 64.0%-77.6%)."282

The data does not support Lantos and colleagues conclusion that a positive IgM immunoblot led to diagnostic uncertainty for the doctors at Boston Children's Hospital. "A false positive IgM immunoblot may lead to diagnostic uncertainty and the potential for over-diagnosis of Lyme disease." concludes Lantos.[282] Over 70 percent of children with a positive IgM immunoblot had Lyme disease by the authors by their restrictive definition. Moreover, the authors dismissed the possibility that children admitted to Boston Children's Hospital with nonspecific clinical presentations or ill for more than two months could indeed have had Lyme disease.

The data also failed to recognize that doctor's at Boston Children's Hospital use clinical judgment when admitting children with a positive IgM immunoblot in their conclusion. "Clinicians should only obtain Lyme testing in children with a clinical constellation consistent with potential Lyme disease. A positive IgM immunoblot test result alone should be interpreted with caution to avoid Lyme disease over-diagnosis."

Lantos and colleagues did not appear to consider that the patients admitted to Boston Children's Hospital with a positive IgM western blot that did not progress to a positive IgG western blot may, in fact, have had Lyme disease.

IN NEED OF A BETTER UNDERSTANDING OF LYME DISEASE IN CHILDREN

Steere and colleagues describe an epidemic of oligoarticular arthritis in children and adults in three Connecticut communities. "Attacks were usually short (median 1 week) with much longer intervening periods of complete remission (median 2.5 months), but some attacks lasted for months. To date, the typical patient has had three recurrences, but 16 [of 51] patients had none," say the authors, adding, "Over half had concomitant fever (100° – 103°F), malaise and fatigue, headache, and myalgia."[5]

Only a handful of studies on children and adolescents with tick-borne diseases have been done, despite the prevalence of the diseases in this age group and the potential for long-term health consequences.

Bloom and colleagues from Tufts University School of Medicine in 1998 describe the complications of Lyme disease in children. "Five children [of 86] developed behavioral changes, forgetfulness, declining school performance, headache or fatigue and, in two cases, a partial complex seizure disorder."[21]

Vázquez and colleagues from the Department of Pediatrics and the

Yale Children's Clinical Research Center report children ages 2 to 18 with prior cranial nerve palsy have significantly more behavioral changes (16 percent vs. 2 percent), arthralgias and myalgias (21 percent vs. 5 percent), and memory problems (8 percent vs. 1 percent) an average of four years after treatment for Lyme disease.[22]

CASE STUDY: 7-YEAR-OLD WITH LYME DISEASE PRESENTING AS ADHD

Lyme disease can be difficult to diagnose and treat in children with complex presentations. In 1998, Susan was a 7-year-old girl with a complex presentation described by Fallon and colleagues in a paper titled, "The Underdiagnosis of Neuropsychiatric Lyme Disease in Children and Adults." The paper highlights the importance of correctly diagnosing Lyme disease, as well as the need for follow-ups and re-evaluations. .[178]

In this case, during an initial consult with a neuropsychologist, 7-year-old Susan was diagnosed with attention deficit disorder because she had problems focusing on school work. Yet, she lived in a Lyme endemic area and had an array of other symptoms including:

- lethargy
- irritability
- forgetfulness
- headaches
- poor coordination
- joint pain
- word-finding difficulties

- light and sound sensitivity

According to the authors, "A comprehensive medical work-up, including EEG and MRI were within normal limits, except for a positive Lyme ELISA." Her attention deficit disorder eventually resolved, and her school grades returned to normal following several courses of antibiotics.

However, during "the subsequent 2 years" it appeared that the patient had become "antibiotic-dependent, such that she would do well as long as she stayed on antibiotics and relapse when taken off," write Fallon and colleagues.

"At the age of nine," the researchers wrote, "she was able to come off antibiotics and remained symptom free for three years." During that time, Susan was a student who maintained A grades.

By age 12, however, Susan developed knee pain, frequent headaches, and poor concentration.

"Serologic tests revealed a positive ELISA with fully reactive IgG and IgM Western blots," said the authors. "Treatment with oral cefuroxime for 2 months led to a rapid improvement in all symptoms, however within 2 weeks of stopping antibiotics her symptoms returned."

Her parents and teachers reported numerous other problems:

- They described "trouble with consistency in day-today work; careless; head in the clouds; scattered and sloppy work; assignments are late, forgotten, or lost; difficult time following directions; more forgetful and disorganized."
- "Her parents noted that Susan would go to school with homework in her bag but once there have no idea where it was or whether she had done it."
- "Emotionally, she had become frustrated, overwhelmed,

tearful, aggressive, and fearful with new onset phobias and nightmares."
- "She had knee pain with mild swelling, paresthesias (burning and prickly sensation), headaches, moderate fatigue, insomnia, and trouble focusing."

Her neurocognitive tests revealed she was experiencing problems in six of nine inattention areas which were consistent with attention deficit hyperactivity disorder (ADHD). There was no evidence of depression or suicidal feeling, "but significant deficits in visual motor planning, speed of processing, visual scanning, attention, visual memory, and learning," write Fallon and colleagues.177

Ultimately, Susan was diagnosed as "having a persistent encephalopathy secondary to Lyme disease." After restarting oral cefuroxime, and remaining on the treatment for several months, noted Fallon and colleagues, she eventually returned "to her prior level of health an academic excellence, with no evidence of the prior ADHD symptoms."178

CASE STUDY: 16-YEAR-OLD WITH LYME DISEASE PRESENTING AS DEPRESSION

In a case reported in 1998 by Fallon and colleagues, a 16-year-old boy, named David, was initially presumed to suffer from long-standing depression. He presented with anger, frustration, insomnia, poor appetite, mild weight loss, and passive suicidal ideation." His longstanding depression was "exacerbated recently when he stopped dating a girl after only two weeks because he felt too tired and not smart enough," according to the researchers.[178] "He reported feeling spaced out all the time, as if in a fog." David also lived in a Lyme endemic area.

David's steep decline in cognitive behavior and IQ were initially presumed to be caused by "either laziness or mild depression."

- He quit sports.
- His grades declined from A and A- in seventh grade to nearly failing by tenth grade.
- He appeared lazy because he found it hard to get out of bed in the morning.
- He often forgot to hand in assignments that he had in fact completed.

- He reported trouble staying awake in class and trouble concentrating.

His symptoms were extensive:

- severe headaches
- facial fasciculations (muscle twitches),
- myalgias
- stiff neck
- hyperacusis (sensitivity to sounds)
- episodic paresthesias (burning or prickling sensation) of his face and hands
- sudden sweating
- painful joints
- sore throats
- palpitations
- electric-shock-like pains
- word-finding problems such that it was hard to finish sentences
- semantic paraphasias
- short-term memory problems such that he could not recall conversations
- testicular pain

While the young man had "had embedded tick bites," wrote the researchers, "he could not recall ever having had an erythema migrans rash."

David's "Lyme ELISA was negative twice in the prior 3 months, his IgG Western blot revealed 4 of the 5 requisite CDC specific bands." The neuropsychologic evaluation, said the researchers, showed "significant deficits in processing speed and visual spatial memory." Researchers added, testing by a brain SPECT "revealed moderate to severe diffusely and heterogeneously decreased perfusion in the cortex and the central white matter, consistent with encephalitis, vasculitis, and Lyme disease."

David was diagnosed and treated with excellent results for probable Lyme encephalopathy with 12 weeks of intravenous ceftriaxone. He improved on sleep, appetite, headaches, joint pains, numbness, distractibility, short-term memory, and emotional behavior. His depression cleared without the need for antidepressant medications. His IQ improved by 22 points, and his school performance markedly improved.

Like the case of 7-year-old Susan, David's case also illustrates the need for careful diagnosis and treatment of tick-borne infections in young people. So often these infections look like the common problems see in school-aged children: depression, ADHD, joint pains from growth spurts. These cases show the need to not only look at symptoms, but to be mindful of where students live and play.

CHILDREN TESTING POSITIVE FOR BABESIA MICROTI

The high prevalence of Babesia found in serum samples is not new. A 2016 study published in *Vector-Borne and Zoonotic Diseases* found that 28.6 percent of serum samples taken from individuals with Lyme disease tested positive for Babesia.[61]

"Reported co-infection rates of *B. microti* with *B. burgdorferi* in humans vary greatly and can range from 10 percent to 32 percent,"[60,283] according to Curcio and colleagues from the Department of Biomedical Sciences, Long Island University.[61] Diuk-Wasser and colleagues report that up to 40 percent of patients with Lyme disease experienced concurrent babesiosis, in the 2015 issue of *Trends in Parasitology*.[58]

Of children included in the Curcio study, half of those ages 2 to 10 with serologic evidence of a tick-borne illness tested positive for Babesia. Of those ages 11 to 20 with serologic evidence of a tick-borne illness, four of 11 tested positive for Babesia.[61]

Identifying Babesia is critical because antibiotic treatment differs from that prescribed for Lyme disease. "Doxycycline is the preferred oral treatment because it has activity against other tick-borne illnesses such as human granulocytic anaplasmosis, whereas the treatment for babesiosis is a combination of atovaquone and azithromycin," explain Curcio and colleagues.[61]

Unfortunately, doctors may not be ordering tests for Babesia. Only 3 percent of nearly 3 million Lyme patients from seven large commercial laboratories were tested for Babesia.[142] In other words, only 85,323 Babesia tests were ordered compared with more than 2 million Lyme disease tests.

CASE STUDY: 10-YEAR-OLD BOY WITH LYME DISEASE IN INDIA

*D*octors have been looking for Lyme disease cases since first described 40 years ago by Steere and colleagues in the Lyme, Conn., area of the United States. The disease has since been confirmed as far away as India.

Doctors describe acute Lyme disease in a 10-year-old boy from Himachal Pradesh, a nonendemic area in India, in the 2017 *Indian Dermatology Online Journal*. The boy developed a rash following a trip to a nearby forest. The rash was described as an Erythematous annular plaque measuring approximately 6 by 5 cm with a central blister on the back of the left leg. "Clinical diagnosis of erythema chronica migrans (ECM) was made," according to Sharma and colleagues from the Departments of Dermatology and Paediatrics, Regional Hospital, Bilaspur, India.[284]

Laboratory evidence was supportive, but the western blot was not done because of financial constraints. Serology for *Borrelia burgdorferi* Ospc (23 KDa) antigen was done with the enzyme-immunoassay technique. IgM was raised at 4.4 U/ml (normal less than 0.90) using serology for *B. burgdorferi* Outer surface protein C (Ospc) (23 KDa) antigen. "Biopsy from the active margin of the lesion showed moderate perivascular lymphocytic infiltrate with a focus of spongiosis, with papillary dermis showing extravasation of red blood cells," according to Sharma and colleagues.[284]

The lesion resolved with three weeks of doxycycline.

The authors list other reports of Lyme disease in India in the literature. "This case report highlights the possibility of future risk of Lyme disease in Himachal Pradesh and warrants the treating physicians to be aware of its occurrence in this part of the world," note Sharma and colleagues.[284]

The authors' observations will no likely be questioned, just as they would be in the United States. Nevertheless, their case reminds us of the need for further study.

SECTION XI. EDUCATION AND PREVENTION

What makes ticks tick? With the explosion of tick-borne diseases in the United States and worldwide, researchers have been learning more and more about tick behavior and what we can do to prevent infection. The following discussions address practical questions: How easy is it to pick up a questing tick? How long must a tick be attached to infect you? Can ticks jump from your dog to you? How do you kill a tick? And plenty more intriguing topics.

HALF OF CONNECTICUT FAMILIES HAVE HAD AT LEAST ONE MEMBER WITH A TICKBORNE DISEASE

The number of Connecticut residents who have a history of a tick-borne illness is overwhelming. According to a 2014 survey, published in *Ticks and Tick-borne Diseases*, 30 percent of the residents sampled had received treatment for a tick-transmitted illness, while 50 percent reported another family member having had a tick-borne disease.[197]

The survey's data should not come as a surprise. In 2004, while testifying before the Connecticut Public Health Department, the state's chief epidemiologist, Dr. James Hadler, warned officials that "roughly 1 percent of the entire population, or probably 34,000 people, are getting a diagnosis of Lyme disease in Connecticut each year." He explained that meant 20 percent to 25 percent of all families in the state had at least one person diagnosed with Lyme disease, and 3 percent to 5 percent of all families had someone diagnosed with Lyme disease in the previous year.[285]

In the years since Hadler's testimony, Lyme disease has escalated far beyond a mere blip on the radar. The complexity of the Lyme spirochete, the difficulty in diagnosing and treating the infection, the growing number of cases, and the spread of the disease into new geographic regions within the United States and worldwide, have elevated Lyme disease to a whole new level.

HOW EASY IS IT TO PICK UP A QUESTING TICK? PRETTY EASY.

*H*ow concerned should you be about ticks getting on your clothes, biting you, and causing Lyme disease or other tick-borne infections? What are the odds that a tick has attached itself to your socks, pant legs, or shirt while you were enjoying the great outdoors? Nelson and colleagues, in the journal *Ticks and Tick-Borne Diseases*, cite two studies that answer those questions.[286] And the odds are in favor of the tick.

"In one Maryland study, an investigator simulated outdoor activities such as gardening or clearing brush by crawling through leaf litter for 30-second time periods. *I. scapularis* nymphs were acquired in 58 percent of crawls, and the majority of ticks were found on pant legs and socks."[287]

The authors note that in another study, "investigators who walked a series of 100 meter transects through a wooded area in New Jersey found an average of nine *I. scapularis* adults on their clothing afterward."[288]

HOW LONG MUST A TICK BE ATTACHED TO TRANSMIT LYME BACTERIA?

How long must a tick be attached to transmit the Lyme bacteria to an individual? Is it 48 hours, 36 hours, 24 or less?

Michael J Cook, an independent researcher, Dorset, U.K., explores the topic in a 2014 article titled "Lyme Borreliosis: A Review of Data on Transmission Time After Tick Attachment" in the *International Journal of Internal Medicine*. "It is frequently stated that the risk of infection is very low if the tick is removed within 24 to 48 hours with some claims that there is no risk if an attached tick is removed within 24 hours or 48 hours."[278]

According to Cook, those claims "are not supported by the published data, and the minimum tick attachment time for transmission in humans has never been established."[278]

He notes that "a literature review has determined that in animal models, transmission can occur in less than 16 hours, and the minimum attachment time for transmission of infection has never been established. No studies have been carried out to characterize transmission with attachment times of less than 16 hours and some did not report any data for less than 36 hours."

For now, many public health agencies, including the Centers for Disease Control and Prevention (CDC), assure the public that most ticks "must be attached for 36 to 48 hours or more before the Lyme disease bacterium can be transmitted."[289]

The literature review by Cook summarizes the shortcomings of the evidence on how long a tick must be attached to transmit Lyme bacteria to an individual.

PARTIALLY FED TICKS CAN REATTACH TO A SECOND HOST AND FEED

Many people mistakenly believe that once a tick attaches, it will remain attached throughout its entire feeding or until it is removed. But that isn't the case. In a 1993 mouse study, researchers found that ticks can spontaneously detach during the feeding process.[290]

"We found that nymphs do detach spontaneously from free-ranging mice in the laboratory, perhaps as frequently as 15 percent of the time," reports Shih and colleagues from the Department of Tropical Public Health, Harvard School of Public Health, Boston, Mass. "Indeed, about [one tenth] of questing nymphs in nature seem to be distended, and reattachment by partially fed sub-adult ticks commonly occurs."[290]

In the laboratory, partially fed ticks would reattach to a second host and commence feeding. According to Shih and colleagues, "Virtually all nymphal ticks that previously had fed for 16 hours reattached efficiently."[290]

In a partially fed tick, spirochetes multiply in the mid-gut and then move to the salivary glands. If the tick bites again, the spirochetes residing in the salivary glands can be transmitted more quickly. "Partially fed nymphs [ticks] are able to reattach to another host," according to the authors. "Lyme disease spirochetes may be transmitted by partially fed nymphs more rapidly than by nymphs that have not already fed."[290]

These findings are particularly relevant to people who own pets. "These partially fed ticks may already have acquired spirochetal infection and avidly seek other hosts," say Shih and colleagues. "Pet ownership appears to be a risk factor for human Lyme disease, and this may reflect contact with ticks that have detached from a cat or dog within the household."[85]

SIX MINUTES IN YOUR CLOTHES DRYER WILL KILL A TICK

The quickest way to kill a tick on clothes is to throw the clothes directly in the dryer before washing them. That's the finding of Nelson and colleagues from the Centers for Disease Control and Prevention (CDC). Standard-sized, residential washers and dryers were used in the study.

"Placing clothing directly in a dryer and drying for a minimum of six minutes on high heat will effectively kill ticks on clothing," report the authors.

It takes much longer to kill a tick in your washer. "If clothing is soiled and requires washing first, our results indicate clothing should be washed with water temperature [equal to or greater than] 54°C (130°F) to kill ticks," report Nelson and colleagues. It was more difficult to kill nymphal and adult ticks at lower temperatures. The authors report that half of the ticks survived hot-water washes when the water temperature was less than 54°C (130°F).

So, while warm- or cold-water washes may be gentler on your clothes, they allow ticks to live on. "The majority (94 percent) of ticks survived warm washes [temperature range between 27° and 46°C (80°

and 115°F)] and all ticks survived cold washes [15° to 27°C (59° to 80°F)]."

If ticks survive a wash cycle, it's still possible to kill them in the dryer. But the temperature must be even higher. "When subsequently dried on a high heat setting [54° to 85°C (129° to 185°F)], it took 50 minutes to kill all ticks (95 percent confidence limit)."

Nelson and colleagues point out that most nymphal ticks did not survive beyond 30 minutes of drying time. Only one tick was found to survive at 40 minutes and had died before it was rechecked at 50 minutes.

The authors don't identify additional factors that may have contributed to killing the ticks, such as the effects of detergents or dryer sheets. Furthermore, they warn, killing other types of ticks might be more difficult. "For example, *Amblyomma americanum* ticks (also known as lone star ticks) are more resistant to low humidity and would potentially survive longer in dryers."[286]

"Following each wash and dry cycle, tick survival was assessed by observing the ticks for normal behavior and movement," say Nelson and colleagues. "If ticks appeared to be moribund and movement was not readily apparent, ticks were lightly probed with forceps, exposed to carbon dioxide through exhalation, and observed for several additional minutes."

The authors say that to verify that motionless ticks were in fact dead and not simply stunned, they "were then placed in petri dishes with a piece of wet paper towel and reassessed 20 to 24 hours later."[286]

Our takeaway from this long-overdue study by the CDC is to dry first at high heat, wash later. And skip the cold-water washes. They may preserve your clothes but not necessarily your health.

RISK OF A TICK BITE HIGHER FOR PET OWNERS

Are pet owners more at risk of being bitten by a tick? Yes, according to a study in the journal *Zoonoses Public Health*.[338] The risk is significantly higher for both dog and cat owners. Jones and colleagues looked at 2,727 households in three Lyme disease endemic states. More than half (56.7 percent) reported owning at least one indoor-outdoor pet, either a dog or cat, or both.

Of 1,546 households with pets, 88.1 percent used some form of tick control on their pets. Yet 20 percent still found ticks on their pets, 31.4 percent reported ticks crawling on family members, and 19.2 percent found ticks attached to family members during the study period, according to Jones and colleagues from the Maryland Department of Health and Mental Hygiene, Baltimore, Md.[338]

Overall, pet-owning households reportedly had a 1.83 times greater risk of finding ticks crawling on family members and a 1.49 times greater risk of having attached ticks.[338]

For those households that found ticks on their pets, the risk of a human-and-tick encounter increased significantly, with a 2.69 times greater risk of a tick crawling on a family member and a 2.5 greater risk of tick attachment. "We were surprised," say the authors, "to find that the reported use of tick control on pets did not have a protective effect on tick encounters."[338]

The authors also found that certain property features increased the likelihood of human-and-tick encounters. Homes with a vegetable garden, compost pile, log pile, bird feeder, stone walls, and children's play equipment were at a greater risk of "finding ticks both crawling and attached to household members."[338]

There may be several reasons why the risk of tick exposure is greater for pet owners. The authors suggest:[338]

1. Pets may bring ticks onto the property and even into the home, where humans can encounter them.
2. Pet owners may engage in activities with their pets that take both themselves and their pets into tick habitat, increasing the risk of tick encounters.
3. Pet ownership is increasing in the United States, and many pet owners allow their pets to share their living space, including furniture and beds.

This study did not demonstrate an association between tick encounters in pet-owning households and tick-borne diseases. However, another analysis found "self-reported tick encounters may be a robust surrogate for disease risk at the household level." According to the authors, "The greater risk of encountering ticks in pet-owning households reflects a true increase in risk of tick-borne disease in these households."[338]

Pet owners should be made aware of these risks and reminded to conduct tick checks regularly on pets and household members. They also should consult their veterinarian regarding effective tick-control products.

TICKS BITE DURING WINTER MONTHS IN THE SOUTH

Tick bite during the warmer months in the North. Ticks don't typically bite during the winter months in the northeastern United States except during a warm spell.

In contrast, ticks bite during the winter months in the South when the weather is more moderate. However, "A 10-year Study of Tick Biting in Mississippi," published in 2008, found the majority of bites by *Ixodes scapularis* deer ticks occur during the winter months in the South.[291]

To identify the types of ticks biting Mississippi residents, researchers collected 119 ticks from 73 people over a 10-year-period. They identified seven tick species and discovered that the lone star species was the most likely to bite individuals in Mississippi, accounting for 52.9 percent of the reported tick bites.

The gulf coast tick was the second-most common, followed by the American dog tick and the *I. scapularis*.[291] The *I. scapularis* ticks were only found from November to April.

LARVAL TICKS A THREAT WITH THE DISCOVERY OF B. MIYAMOTOI

Tiny larval ticks previously have not been considered a threat to humans. Experts long believed that an adult female tick could not pass on any infections to the eggs and larvae. As a result, ticks in the larva stage were thought to be free from carrying diseases and therefore harmless. But that may not be so, according to a case series by Molloy and colleagues published in 2015 in the *Annals of Internal Medicine*.[65]

When ticks hatch from eggs, they're called larvae. At this stage, they have only six legs. After taking their first blood meal, the larvae molt into 8-legged nymphal ticks. Most studies have identified black-legged ticks in the nymph stage as posing the greatest threat to humans. But Molloy and colleagues now raise concerns that newly hatched larvae, which are microscopic in size, may be just as dangerous.[65]

While investigating the clinical spectrum and effectiveness of laboratory testing for *Borrelia miyamotoi* disease, one of the newer tick-borne infections, Molloy and colleagues found that most cases occurred in July and August. Those are the months when larvae ticks are most active. Nymphal ticks, in contrast, are most abundant in June and early July.

The timing of *B. miyamotoi* peak incidence in the case series was consistent with transovarial transmission described in 2001 by Scoles and colleagues, Yale University School of Medicine[292] "Transovarial transmission was demonstrated by PCR of larval progeny from infected females, with filial infection rates ranging from 6 percent to 73 percent," according to the authors.[292]

"Bites from larval deer ticks have not been considered a health threat, but this needs to be reevaluated," write Krause from the Yale School of Public Health and Barbour from the University of California – Irvine, in an accompanying editorial.[293]

LARVAL TICKS MAY BE A THREAT TO HUMANS AFTER ALL

Researchers found that larvae of *Ixodes ricinus* can transmit *Borrelia afzelii* and *Borrelia miyamotoi* to rodents.[294] Their 2016 paper was published in *Parasites & Vectors*. The authors estimate that individuals living in the Netherlands receive at least 30,000 larval bites out of 1.1 million tick bites annually.

Larval bites of humans, which easily go unnoticed, can cause *Lyme borreliosis* and *B. miyamotoi* disease," according to van Duijvendijk and colleagues from the Laboratory of Entomology, Wageningen University, The Netherlands.

The authors of the study suggest that patients who do not report seeing a tick bite may acquire *Lyme borreliosis* from the bite of a larval tick. Its minute size makes it easy to overlook, and it has now been shown to transmit the disease.

"Larval transmission of *B. miyamotoi* has implications for checking for ticks and continuing tick precautions even after the risk of Lyme disease has abated," say Krause and colleagues from Yale University School of Public Health.[12]

The authors conclude, "This finding changes the current view on the enzootic lifecycle of *B. afzelii* and the current public health dogma that larval bites cannot cause Lyme disease in humans."

PERMETHRIN-TREATED CLOTHING CAUSES 'HOT FOOT' EFFECT IN TICKS

Numerous studies have found that wearing permethrin-treated clothing can reduce the risk of tick bites. A University of Rhode Island study found that people wearing permethrin-treated sneakers and socks were 73.6 times less likely to be bitten by a tick than those wearing untreated footwear.[356] But very few studies have looked at the behavior of a tick when it comes in contact with permethrin-treated clothing. Does it climb onto the insecticide-soaked textile or avoid it entirely? Does permethrin actually kill ticks?

Scientists treated a model that mimicked a pant leg or the arm of a long-sleeved shirt with permethrin, then studied the behavior and fate of ticks when exposed to the clothing. The findings were reported in the journal *Ticks and Tick-borne Diseases*.[357]

"permethrin-treated textiles did not repel ticks without contact, as seen with DEET." according to Eisen and colleagues from the Division of Vector-Borne Diseases, National Center for Emerging and Zoonotic Infectious Diseases at the Centers for Disease Control and Prevention in Colorado.[357] In fact, the majority (88 percent) of nymphal ticks chose to move onto permethrin-treated textile but not DEET-treated textile.

After coming in contact with the treated clothing, the ticks dislodged through a "hot-foot" effect. "Ticks readily walked onto a permethrin-treated textile," say the authors. But the "laboratory-reared ticks became visibly agitated, displaying a hot-foot effect, and escaped contact with the permethrin-treated textile by tumbling downwards until they dislodged themselves completely from a textile-covered assay card."[357]

However, field-collected ticks were hardier than laboratory-reared ticks, and they could sustain longer contact with the treated textile. The authors postulate that field-collected ticks have been exposed to highly variable temperatures and humidity, which may result in slower absorption of permethrin. "However, by 1- and 24-hours post-exposure, very few ticks displayed normal movement, thus presenting minimal risk to bite, regardless of whether they were reared in the laboratory or collected in the field."[357]

"Contact with permethrin-treated textiles negatively impacts the vigor and behavior of nymphal ticks for [more than] 24 hours, with outcomes ranging from complete lack of movement to impaired movement and unwillingness of ticks displaying normal movement to ascend onto a human finger," according to the authors.[357]

One day after exposure, most ticks were completely motionless. The remaining ticks could recover. "Ticks having recovered normal movement 1 day after exposure in our study most often ascended onto a finger when given the opportunity (and presumably also were capable of biting)," the authors point out. In a real-life scenario, the ticks that fall off will likely die over time.[357]

In real life, a tick may walk underneath the treated textile such as permethrin treated shorts or a T-shirt.[357]

Permethrin is acutely toxic in high doses. The authors did not address the potential toxicity of permethrin to humans. "Acute signs of toxicity to the central nervous system include incoordination, ataxia, hyperactivity, convulsions, and finally prostration, paralysis, and death," according to a review by the National Research Council (US) Subcommittee to Review Permethrin Toxicity from Military Uniforms.[358] [3] Users have been advised not to inhale permethrin when treating cloths and not to apply permethrin to the skin.

LACK OF AWARENESS OF BABESIA AND ANAPLASMOSIS

A 2014 survey of Connecticut residents found that surprisingly few people living in the Lyme-endemic southwestern region of the state were aware of Babesia. And, even fewer were familiar with *Anaplasmosis*. The results were published in a 2015 issue of *Ticks and Tick-borne Diseases*.[197]

Only 23 percent of 275 people surveyed living in the southwestern region of Connecticut were aware that deer ticks could transmit Babesia. Only 12 percent of them knew deer ticks could transmit *Anaplasmosis*.

It's common to find ticks and enzootic hosts carrying more than one illness. In fact, between 12 percent and 42 percent of rodents are coinfected with both *Borrelia burgdorferi* (the cause of Lyme disease) and *Babesia microti*. Up to 40 percent of patients with Lyme disease experience concurrent babesiosis.[58]

It's important for doctors and their patients to be aware of co-infections.

SECTION XII. RESEARCH AND NOVEL APPROACHES

Researchers continue to study how our body systems respond to the pathogens set loose by the bite of a tick. Why does the immune system respond as it does to early Lyme disease? Why does the brain exaggerate responses to painful stimuli in some patients? Can the speed of Lyme bacteria be slowed down? These discussions concern research at the very forefront of medical science, and could eventually lead to a cure.

WHAT COULD HAPPEN TO THE BRAIN DURING ACUTE INFECTION?

*P*atients diagnosed with Lyme neuroborreliosis typically suffer from headaches, fatigue, memory loss, learning disabilities, and depression. Clinical findings have included meningitis, cranial neuritis, encephalopathy, encephalitis, encephalomyelitis, radiculitis, radiculoneuritis, mononeuropathies, plexopathies, and demyelinating neuropathies.

Philipp and colleagues at the Tulane National Primate Research Center[295] examined the role of inflammation on the central nervous system of subjects infected with *Borrelia burgdorferi.* Rhesus monkeys were injected with live *B. burgdorferi* spirochete. Several monkeys received a potent steroid prior to being injected with the spirochete, while another group was pretreated with a non-steroidal anti-inflammatory drug (NSAID).

The NSAID group and the control group both experienced extensive neurologic damage. The monkeys' cerebrospinal fluid revealed significantly elevated levels of IL-6, IL-8, chemokine ligand 2, CXCL13, and pleocytosis, according to a study published in *The American Journal of Pathology.*[296]

Pathological changes included:

1. leptomeningitis (meningitis)
2. vasculitis (inflammation of blood vessels in the brain)
3. focal inflammation in the central nervous system
4. necrotizing focal myelitis in the cervical spinal cord
5. radiculitis (pain that radiates along the nerve due to inflammation on the nerve root at its connection to the spinal column)
6. neuritis (inflammation of the nerves)
7. demyelination in the spinal roots (erosion of the myelin sheath that normally protects nerve fibers)
8. inflammation with neurodegeneration in the dorsal root ganglia (inflammation and progressive loss of structure or function of neurons in the dorsal root ganglia, or spinal ganglion; the dorsal root ganglion contains the cell bodies of sensory neurons that bring information from the periphery to the spinal cord)
9. neuronal and satellite glial cell apoptosis
10. persistent abnormal F-wave chrono dispersions localized to the nerve roots, suggesting damage to axons or demyelination similar to those of several inflammatory demyelinating peripheral neuropathic disorders, including Guillain-Barré syndrome (a rare disorder in which your body's immune system attacks your nerves)

The researchers could prevent the inflammation if the monkeys were pretreated with the potent steroid dexamethasone, but not with non-steroidal medications.

While the monkey study provides insight into the benefits steroids can play when inflammation is present, it's not practical to take steroids prior to a tick bite. Clinicians should not prescribe steroids to patients suspected of having Lyme disease based on this primate study. Rather, they must continue to search out other ways to control the immune response to Lyme disease.

What this study does show is the debilitating consequences some people infected with Lyme disease could potentially face.

T-CELL CHEMOKINE LEVELS CAN REMAIN HIGH IN LYME DISEASE

T-cell chemokines are an important part of the body's immune response in early Lyme disease according to researchers from Johns Hopkins School of Medicine. In fact, Aucott and colleagues specifically identified CCL19 T-cell chemokines in this process. The CCL19 T-cell chemokines rise in early Lyme disease only to drop to normal in 86 percent of patients following treatment with a three-week course of antibiotics. [130]

In a clinical cohort study by the researchers, the T-cell CCL19 chemokines remained high in the 14 percent of Lyme disease patients with Post Treatment Lyme Disease Syndrome. The levels were 12 times higher than normal a month after treatment, note the researchers.[130]

Additional studies have identified the elevation of chemokine CCL19 in the cerebrospinal fluid (CSF) of patients with inflammatory neurological diseases and multiple sclerosis (MS).[297] Another identified chemokine, CXCL13, was also elevated in the CSF of patients with MS, neuroborreliosis, and other inflammatory neurological diseases.[297]

Chemokine elevations have been seen in other autoimmune conditions as well, including in the liver during chronic hepatitis C infection, the synovium in rheumatoid arthritis, and the salivary glands in Sjogren's syndrome.

Researchers continue to look at what causes the elevation of CCL19 chemokine levels. Aucott and colleagues hypothesize one answer could be an ongoing immune-driven reaction to an ongoing infection.[130]

THE BRAIN HAS EXAGGERATED RESPONSES TO PAIN AND NON-PAINFUL STIMULI

The value of a well-designed, peer-reviewed research study can often be seen in the studies it spawns in other disciplines. In the case of Lyme disease, researchers have learned patients with Lyme disease experience exaggerated responses to pain and non-painful stimuli despite antibiotic treatment.[298,299] Understanding why Lyme disease patients have those responses might be answered, in part, by a 2017 study by Lopez-Sola and colleagues.

In that study, by Lopez-Sola et.al., measured the brain's response to pain and non-painful stimuli in fibromyalgia patients. The methodology from this study, and the ultimate findings, suggest those same pain and non-painful stimuli can be measured in patients with Lyme disease.

"In addition to pain-related changes," the authors pointed out, "fibromyalgia patients show reduced tolerance (augmented unpleasantness) to non-painful sensory stimulation (visual, auditory, olfactory, and tactile), along with abnormal brain processing of nonpainful sensory stimuli."[300] Their findings were reported in 2016 in the journal *PAIN*, published by the International Association for the Study of Pain.

Lopez-Sola's team used Functional Magnetic Resonance Imaging (fMRI) to demonstrate an exaggerated response to pain and nonpainful stimuli in fibromyalgia patients. The fMRI has previously been used to measure regional, time-varying changes in the brain's metabolism as a biomarker for disease and to monitor therapy, and also for studying pharmacological efficacy.[301]

The team exposed 37 fibromyalgia patients and 35 control patients to painful pressure. "When the people with fibromyalgia were exposed to the painful stimuli, they had greater Neurologic Pain Signature (NPS) responses than those without the condition."

Greater responses were also described for non-painful visual, auditory, and tactile stimuli. "In fibromyalgia, the misfiring and irregular engagement of different parts of the brain to process normal sensory stimuli like light, sound, pressure, temperature, and odor results in pain, flu-like sensations, or other symptoms.

"This extra brain work can be exhausting," explains Jan Chambers, founder of the National Fibromyalgia & Chronic Pain Association.[302]

"The potential for brain measures like the ones we developed here is that they can tell us something about the particular brain abnormalities that drive an individual's suffering," states Wager, director of the Cognitive and Affective Control Laboratory, University of Colorado Boulder.[303]

The fMRI can provide clinicians with insight into the neural pathology underlying fibromyalgia pain symptoms. According to Lopez-Sola and colleagues, "The novelty of this study is that it provides potential neuroimaging-based tools that can be used with new patients to inform about the degree of certain neural pathology underlying their pain symptoms."[302]

The fMRI results may also help predict treatment responses in fibromyalgia by establishing "a framework for assessing therapeutic mechanisms and predicting treatment response at the individual level," the authors say.

"The brain changes due to pain consisted of augmented responses in sensory integration (insula/operculum) and self-referential (e.g., medial prefrontal) regions in fibromyalgia, and reduced responses in the lateral frontal cortex," describe Lopez-Sola and colleagues. "The brain changes due to non-painful sensory stimulation consisted of augmented responses in insula/operculum, posterior cingulate, and medial prefrontal regions, and reduced responses in primary/secondary sensory cortices, basal ganglia, and cerebellum."

The authors caution that exaggerated responses to pain and non-painful stimuli are not unique to fibromyalgia. "Notably, we do not imply that the signature should differentiate fibromyalgia from other chronic pain conditions with a sensitization component."

The exaggerated response to pain and non-painful stimuli described in their fibromyalgia patients could explain the exaggerated responses to pain and non-painful stimuli seen in patients with tick-borne illnesses such as Lyme disease.

NEW TOOLS MIGHT VALIDATE BRAIN'S EXAGGERATED RESPONSE TO SENSORY INPUT

*L*yme disease patients frequently report central sensitization or sensory hyperarousal. In patients with Post-Treatment Lyme Disease Syndrome (PTLSD), "sensory hyperarousal was reported by a majority of patients after acquiring Lyme disease, most often affecting hearing and/or vision," according to Batheja and colleagues from the Department of Psychiatry, Columbia University.[298]

"Hypersensitivity to sound may be limited to louder sounds, but, in some individuals, even the volume fluctuations in a normal conversation can be noxious," according to Batheja and colleagues.[298] "These patients might be seen wearing earplugs or sound-protectors when in situations normally tolerable to others."

They add, "The individual's life may be quite altered by this hypersensitivity: wearing sunglasses indoors and avoidance of being outside during daylight, which, in turn, limits the ability to sustain a normal work and social life."[298]

Hypersensitivity in other sensory modalities, such as olfactory, tactile, gustatory, and temperature, have been described, according to Batheja and colleagues.[298] Hypersensitivity to sound has also been described elsewhere.[304]

Acute and chronic pain associated with Lyme borreliosis has been characterized as having "qualities of neuropathic pain, that is, radicular, deep aching, or lancinating pain, often worse at night, and associated with both sensory and motor findings," according to Zimering and colleagues.[299] "Chronic pain despite adequate antibiotic treatment of neuroborreliosis was reported by a substantial number of patients described by various investigators."[299]

A team of researchers in Colorado demonstrated the effectiveness of using neuroimaging-based tools to help validate pain symptoms and gauge treatment response in patients with fibromyalgia.[300]

The same neuroimaging-based tools could help validate pain and nonpainful stimuli and gauge treatment response in patients with Lyme disease.

ACTIVATED ASTROCYTES COULD LEAD TO LONG-TERM BRAIN INJURY

A study by Casselli and colleagues found that *Borrelia burgdorferi* activates human astrocytes cells in culture. Astrocytes are cells found in abundance in the central nervous system (CNS) that have been described as "key responders to CNS infection and important components of the blood-brain barrier," in the journal *PLoS One*.[305]

"If uncontrolled in the context of neuroborreliosis, the astrocyte response could lead to long-term injury in the CNS,"[305] according to Casselli and colleagues from the Department of Biomedical Sciences, University of North Dakota School of Medicine and Health Sciences.

"Understanding how these changes are maintained over time will be of great importance in developing effective treatments [for] Lyme disease," according to the authors. "The pathophysiology behind the neurocognitive complaints of Lyme disease is unclear, but the inflammatory response to the bacterium or its components is likely to play a role."

OVER-SHOOTING B CELL RESPONSE MAY CONTRIBUTE TO BRAIN PATHOLOGY

A study examined why 23 of 77 patients with Lyme neuroborreliosis suffered from ongoing illness despite treatment.

These 23 patients had higher levels of the Th17-associated markers (IL-17A) and the B cell associated markers (CXCL13, APRIL, and BAFF) in their spinal fluid than did controls.[306]

"Speculatively, moderate levels reflect an appropriate B cell response, while higher levels may reflect an over-shooting response mirroring or even contributing to more extensive CNS [central nervous system] pathology," explain Gyllemark and colleagues in the *Journal of Neuroinflammation*.

The authors did not address whether a persistent infection might explain the persistently high levels of B cell response because the study was retrospective.

SLOWING DOWN THE LYME DISEASE SPIROCHETE

The Lyme disease bacterium swims in an undulating pattern throughout the body. "The flagella reside within the periplasm, the space between the bacterial cell wall and the outer membrane," according to Harman and colleagues from the Department of Molecular and Cellular Biology, University of Arizona.[307] "Rotation of the flagella within the periplasm causes the waveform to propagate, leading to a traveling wave undulation of the entire body."

The researchers' earlier work with mathematical modeling predicted that the shape of a Lyme disease spirochete might impact pathogenesis. "Consequently, altering the shape and/or stiffness of the bacterium could affect pathogenesis," say Harman and colleagues.[307]

The antibiotic Vancomycin reportedly reduced the swimming speed of the Lyme disease spirochete by about 15 percent by reducing the cell wall stiffness, according to Harman.[307]

The authors conclude that "since motility is crucial to the virulence of *B. burgdorferi*, the results suggest that sublethal doses of antibiotics could negatively impact spirochete survival by impeding their swim speed, thereby enabling their capture and elimination by phagocytes."[307]

Their conclusions are based on *in vitro* laboratory data. It is not clear if findings in the lab can be generalized to humans. Moreover, it is not clear if vancomycin would be the best approach. The medical community has sought to limit the use of the drug to fighting severe infections such as MRSA (methicillin-resistant staphylococcus aureus) and penicillin-resistant pneumococci.[308]

PERSISTER CELLS MAY COMPLICATE TREATMENT

Some doctors have concluded that a short course of antibiotics will cure Lyme disease infection, but studies indicate otherwise. Persistent infection of *Borrelia burgdorferi* has been proven experimentally in Peromyscus mice, laboratory mice, rats, hamsters, gerbils, guinea pigs, dogs, and nonhuman primates.[309-316]

"The main culprit responsible for the tolerance of pathogens to antibiotics is a specialized survivor – a persister," states Hodzic.[317] Since persisters are nongrowing dormant cells, antimicrobials cannot kill them and cannot be cultured. For antibiotics to work effectively, there must be active target cells to attack.

In a study review published in the *Bosnian Journal of Basic Medical Sciences*,[317] Hodzic, of Real-Time PCR Research and Diagnostic Core Facility, School of Veterinary Medicine, University of California, Davis, explores the role "persisters" play in causing chronic Lyme symptoms.

During the course of infection, *B. burgdorferi* proliferates, generating "attenuated," or weakened, spirochetes that have lost one or more small plasmids (small DNA molecules within cells). The attenuated spirochetes remain viable but because of their plasmid loss, they divide slowly. This makes them tolerant of antimicrobials and unable to be cultivated.

"There is clear scientific evidence that a small, heterogeneous subpopulation of surviving spirochetes shows tolerance to antimicrobial agents and can persist in a host for a prolonged period following therapy," says Hodzic.[317]

Further, persisters do not appear immediately. They emerge months after treatment. Hodzic found that noncultivable spirochetes reappeared in the tissues of mice 12 months after antibiotic treatment.[318]

"*B. burgdorferi* is highly prone to plasmid loss[317,319,320] and therefore, plasmid loss is likely to occur during the course of infection and increase over time," Hodzic says. "This may explain why treatment success in humans[70,321] and laboratory mice[322,323] appears to be most effective during early infection."[317]

Persisters also appear in farm and pet animals, insects, rodents, and wild animals, including migratory birds. Selection for antimicrobial resistance/tolerance "can occur anywhere antimicrobial agents are present, the environments most notably sewage and surface," according to Hodzic.[317]

Transmission of antimicrobial resistant/tolerant pathogens of animal origin to humans has been documented for methicillin-resistant *S. aureus*, *E. coli*, Salmonella spp., and Campylobacter spp. Patients might run into a persister before being treated.

The presence of persisters may explain why it is sometimes difficult to find an effective antibiotic to treat Lyme disease patients. Hodzic explains that the antibiotic tolerance in persisters is "likely explained by antimicrobial tolerance (in contrast to antibiotic resistance or inadequate antibiotic treatment), in which all classes of antibiotics fail to completely eliminate non-dividing or slowly dividing subpopulations of a broad array of bacteria and fungi."[317]

COULD DORMANCY ALLOW LYME DISEASE TO SURVIVE ANTIBIOTICS?

"Dormancy is a protective state where diverse bacteria including *M. tuberculosis, S. aureus, T. pallidum* (syphilis), and *B. burgdorferi* (Lyme disease) curtail metabolic activity to survive external stresses, including antibiotics," according to Mali and colleagues from The University of Houston, Department of Biology and Biochemistry, in 2017 in the journal *Bacteriology*.[324]

Feng and colleagues from Johns Hopkins University have been identifying drug candidates from the drug library approved by the Food and Drug Administration that might work on *in vitro B. burgdorferi* persisters.[253]

Persistence may be a subset of dormancy. "Evidence suggests dormancy consists of a continuum of interrelated states including viable but nonculturable (VBNC) and persistence states," according to Mali and colleagues. "VBNC and persistence contribute to antibiotic tolerance, reemergence from latent infections, and even quorum sensing and biofilm formation."

Definitions by Mali and colleagues of persister and VBNC cells offer an insight into dormancy:

- "Persister cells have been identified as a 'small subpopulation of cells that spontaneously enter a dormant, nondividing state,' a definition based on survival after antibiotic treatment of bacterial cell populations."
- VBNC are "living cells that have lost the ability to grow on routine media."

Mali and colleagues acknowledge the difficulties in differentiating and isolating VBNC and persister cells. "Both states exhibit enhanced survival under antibiotic treatment."

Persister and VBNC cells may coexist and may both contribute to reduced metabolic activity, antibiotic tolerance, latent infection, and re-emergence of active infections after resolution of stress, according to the authors.

The authors point out the difference between persister and VBNC as a starting point for discussion:

- "We propose to describe persister cells as proliferation-competent cells that can spontaneously resuscitate after resolution of stress."
- "VBNC cells are induced into a non-proliferative state by external stress and will not resuscitate spontaneously until an appropriate external signal is provided."

The authors' work could lead to identification of proteins that drive the dormant state. These proteins might address the question as to whether dormancy might allow Lyme disease to survive antibiotics.

DOES BORRELIA DNA PERSISTENCE CAUSE PAIN TO PERSIST AFTER LYME 'CURE'?

In an article titled "Doctor Says You Are Cured, But You Still Feel the Pain. Borrelia DNA Persistence in Lyme Disease," Cervantes, from Paul L. Foster School of Medicine, Texas Tech University Health Sciences Center, addresses the persistence of pain as the result of Lyme disease.[345]

Studies indicate that *Borrelia* DNA can persist in animals and humans after antibiotic treatment. Cervantes cites evidence of persistent DNA found up to a year after treatment in the joint fluid of arthritis patients after therapy, in endocardial biopsy specimens from patients with dilated cardiomyopathy, and in the urine of antibiotic-treated patients.[345]

Furthermore, new evidence suggests that persistent bacterial DNA can lead to ongoing symptoms. An antimicrobial peptide (AMP) activates TLR9, an innate immune receptor that leads to type-I interferon production. Such production would translate into symptoms consistent with those typically described by patients suffering from post-treatment Lyme disease syndrome (PTLDS) and explain how illness can persist even in the absence of an active bacterial infection, according to Cervantes.[345]

He encourages attention to the use of DNA-binding AMPs to limit chronic manifestations of Lyme disease. AMPs may also "increase the ability of human macrophages to efficiently remove extracellular spirochetal DNA," Cervantes says.[345]

In the same article, Cervantes raises the question of a persistent infection. "Where is *Borrelia burgdorferi* (*Bb*) hiding from the immune system? *Bb* is an elastic organism, able to modify its morphology to 'swim' in between the fibrous tracts of cartilaginous tissue,"[345] he says.

"Cartilage is a tissue that lacks vasculature, providing the perfect sanctuary for *Bb* to escape from immune cells present in the bloodstream. *Bb* can then remain 'hidden' in the extracellular matrix," he suggests.[345]

Therein lies the $64,000 question: Can persistent *Borrelia* DNA represent a persistent infection? If so, treating a persistent infection with an antibiotic might be more effective than treating with a DNA-binding AMP.

REFERENCES

1. Hesiod, Works and Days from Perseus Digital Library Gregory R. Crane, Editor-in-Chief Tufts University at http://www.perseus.tufts.edu/hopper/text?doc=Perseus%3Atext%3A1999.01.0132%3Acard%3D59. Last accessed 9/25/17.

2. Poinar G, Jr., Brown AE. A new genus of hard ticks in Cretaceous Burmese amber (Acari: Ixodida: Ixodidae). *Syst Parasitol.* 2003;54(3):199-205.

3. Lyme bacterium's possible ancestor found in ancient tick, by Rachel Nuwer, Nature, June 6, 2014. in http://www.nature.com/news/lyme-bacterium-s-possible-ancestor-found-in-ancient-tick-1.15378. Last accessed 3/24/17.

4. Kean WF, Tocchio S, Kean M, Rainsford KD. The musculoskeletal abnormalities of the Similaun Iceman ("OTZI"): clues to chronic pain and possible treatments. *Inflammopharmacology.* 2012.

5. Steere AC, Malawista SE, Snydman DR, et al. Lyme arthritis: an epidemic of oligoarticular arthritis in children and adults in three connecticut communities. *Arthritis Rheum.* 1977;20(1):7-17.

6. Burgdorfer W, Barbour AG, Hayes SF, Benach JL, Grunwaldt E, Davis JP. Lyme disease-a tick-borne spirochetosis? *Science.* 1982;216(4552):1317-1319.

7. Baranton G, Postic D, Saint Girons I, et al. Delineation of Borrelia burgdorferi sensu stricto, Borrelia garinii sp. nov., and group VS461 associated with Lyme borreliosis. *Int J Syst Bacteriol.* 1992;42(3):378-383.

8. Scott JD. Borrelia mayonii: prying open Pandora's box of spirochetes. *Lancet Infect Dis.* 2016;16(6):637.

9. Girard YA, Fedorova N, Lane RS. Genetic diversity of Borrelia burgdorferi and detection of B. bissettii-like DNA in serum of north-coastal California residents. *J Clin Microbiol.* 2011;49(3):945-954.

10. Clark KL, Leydet B, Hartman S. Lyme borreliosis in human patients in Florida and Georgia, USA. *Int J Med Sci.* 2013;10(7):915-931.

11. Rudenko N, Golovchenko M, Vancova M, Clark K, Grubhoffer L, Oliver JH, Jr. Isolation of live Borrelia burgdorferi sensu lato spirochetes from patients with undefined disorders and symptoms not typical for Lyme borreliosis. *Clin Microbiol Infect.* 2015.

12. Krause PJ, Fish D, Narasimhan S, Barbour AG. Borrelia miyamotoi infection in nature and in humans. *Clin Microbiol Infect.* 2015.

13. Krause PJ, Telford SR, 3rd, Ryan R, et al. Geographical and temporal distribution of babesial infection in Connecticut. *J Clin Microbiol.* 1991;29(1):1-4.

14. Dietrich F, Schmidgen T, Maggi RG, et al. Prevalence of Bartonella henselae and Borrelia burgdorferi sensu lato DNA in ixodes ricinus ticks in Europe. *Appl Environ Microbiol.* 2010;76(5):1395-1398.

15. Berghoff W. Chronic Lyme Disease and Co-infections: Differential Diagnosis. *Open Neurol J.* 2012;6:158-178.

16. Logigian EL, Kaplan RF, Steere AC. Chronic neurologic

manifestations of Lyme disease. *N Engl J Med.* 1990;323(21):1438-1444.

17. Fallon BA, Keilp JG, Corbera KM, et al. A randomized, placebo-controlled trial of repeated IV antibiotic therapy for Lyme encephalopathy. *Neurology.* 2008;70(13):992-1003.

18. Fallon BA, Nields JA. Lyme disease: a neuropsychiatric illness. *Am J Psychiatry.* 1994;151(11):1571-1583.

19. Aucott JN, Rebman AW, Crowder LA, Kortte KB. Post-treatment Lyme disease syndrome symptomatology and the impact on life functioning: is there something here? *Qual Life Res.* 2013;22(1):75-84.

20. Klempner MS, Hu LT, Evans J, et al. Two controlled trials of antibiotic treatment in patients with persistent symptoms and a history of Lyme disease. *N Engl J Med.* 2001;345(2):85-92.

21. Bloom BJ, Wyckoff PM, Meissner HC, Steere AC. Neurocognitive abnormalities in children after classic manifestations of Lyme disease. *Pediatr Infect Dis J.* 1998;17(3):189-196.

22. Vazquez M, Sparrow SS, Shapiro ED. Long-term neuropsychologic and health outcomes of children with facial nerve palsy attributable to Lyme disease. *Pediatrics.* 2003;112(2):e93-97.

23. Eisen RJ, Eisen L, Beard CB. County-Scale Distribution of Ixodes scapularis and Ixodes pacificus (Acari: Ixodidae) in the Continental United States. *J Med Entomol.* 2016.

24. Ticks Carry Lyme Disease in Almost Half of U.S. Counties in ScientificAmerican,com by By Lisa Rapaport January 19, 2016 at http://www.scientificamerican.com/article/ticks-carry-lyme-disease-in-almost-half-of-u-s-counties/. Last accessed 7/3/16.

25. Hall JL, Alpers K, Bown KJ, Martin SJ, Birtles RJ. Use of Mass-Participation Outdoor Events to Assess Human Exposure to Tickborne Pathogens. *Emerg Infect Dis.* 2017;23(3):463-467.

26. Robertson JN, Gray JS, Stewart P. Tick bite and Lyme borreliosis

risk at a recreational site in England. *Eur J Epidemiol.* 2000;16(7):647-652.

27. Faulde MK, Rutenfranz M, Hepke J, Rogge M, Gorner A, Keth A. Human tick infestation pattern, tick-bite rate, and associated Borrelia burgdorferi s.l. infection risk during occupational tick exposure at the Seedorf military training area, northwestern Germany. *Ticks Tick Borne Dis.* 2014;5(5):594-599.

28. De Keukeleire M, Vanwambeke SO, Somasse E, Kabamba B, Luyasu V, Robert A. Scouts, forests, and ticks: Impact of landscapes on human-tick contacts. *Ticks Tick Borne Dis.* 2015;6(5):636-644.

29. Hansford KM, Fonville M, Gillingham EL, et al. Ticks and Borrelia in urban and peri-urban green space habitats in a city in southern England. *Ticks Tick Borne Dis.* 2016.

30. Jobe DA, Nelson JA, Adam MD, Martin SA, Jr. Lyme disease in urban areas, Chicago. *Emerg Infect Dis.* 2007;13(11):1799-1800.

31. Jahfari S, Ruyts SC, Frazer-Mendelewska E, Jaarsma R, Verheyen K, Sprong H. Melting pot of tick-borne zoonoses: the European hedgehog contributes to the maintenance of various tick-borne diseases in natural cycles urban and suburban areas. *Parasit Vectors.* 2017;10(1):134.

32. Khatchikian CE, Prusinski MA, Stone M, et al. Recent and rapid population growth and range expansion of the Lyme disease tick vector, Ixodes scapularis, in North America. *Evolution; international journal of organic evolution.* 2015.

33. Ogden NH, Lindsay LR, Hanincova K, et al. Role of migratory birds in introduction and range expansion of Ixodes scapularis ticks and of Borrelia burgdorferi and Anaplasma phagocytophilum in Canada. *Appl Environ Microbiol.* 2008;74(6):1780-1790.

34. Cohen EB, Auckland LD, Marra PP, Hamer SA. Avian Migrants Facilitate Invasions of Neotropical Ticks and Tick-Borne Pathogens into the United States. *Appl Environ Microbiol.* 2015;81(24):8366-8378.

35. DeLuca WV, Woodworth BK, Rimmer CC, et al. Transoceanic migration by a 12 g songbird. *Biol Lett.* 2015;11(4):20141045.

36. Ogden NH, Barker IK, Francis CM, Heagy A, Lindsay LR, Hobson KA. How far north are migrant birds transporting the tick Ixodes scapularis in Canada? Insights from stable hydrogen isotope analyses of feathers. *Ticks Tick Borne Dis.* 2015;6(6):715-720.

37. Koffi JK, Savage J, Thivierge K, et al. Evaluating the submission of digital images as a method of surveillance for Ixodes scapularis ticks. *Parasitology.* 2017:1-7.

38. Madder M, Walker JG, Van Rooyen J, et al. e-Surveillance in animal health: use and evaluation of mobile tools. *Parasitology.* 2012;139(14):1831-1842.

39. Adetunji SA, Krecek RC, Castellanos G, et al. Seroprevalence of Borrelia burgdorferi antibodies in white-tailed deer from Texas. *Int J Parasitol Parasites Wildl.* 2016;5(2):168-174.

40. Feder HM, Jr., Gerber MA, Luger SW, Ryan RW. Persistence of serum antibodies to Borrelia burgdorferi in patients treated for Lyme disease. *Clin Infect Dis.* 1992;15(5):788-793.

41. Tokarz R, Tagliafierro T, Cucura DM, Rochlin I, Sameroff S, Lipkin WI. Detection of Anaplasma phagocytophilum, Babesia microti, Borrelia burgdorferi, Borrelia miyamotoi, and Powassan Virus in Ticks by a Multiplex Real-Time Reverse Transcription-PCR Assay. *mSphere.* 2017;2(2).

42. Levine JF, Apperson CS, Levin M, et al. Stable Transmission of Borrelia burgdorferi Sensu Stricto on the Outer Banks of North Carolina. *Zoonoses Public Health.* 2016.

43. Watson SC, Liu Y, Lund RB, et al. A Bayesian spatio-temporal model for forecasting the prevalence of antibodies to Borrelia burgdorferi, causative agent of Lyme disease, in domestic dogs within the contiguous United States. *PLoS One.* 2017;12(5):e0174428.

44. ESA Position Statement on Tick-Borne Diseases by the The Entomological Society of America (ESA) 7/29/15 at http://www.entsoc.org/PDF/2015/ESA-PolicyStatement-TickBorneDiseases.pdf. Last accessed 3/24/17.

45. Lantos PM, Nigrovic LE, Auwaerter PG, et al. Geographic Expansion of Lyme Disease in the Southeastern United States, 2000-2014. *Open Forum Infect Dis.* 2015;2(4):ofv143.

46. Discover Magazine. The Confounding Debate Over Lyme Disease in the South, December 2013. http://discovermagazine.com/2013/dec/14-southern-gothic. Last accessed 3/24/17.

47. Steere AC, Klitz W, Drouin EE, et al. Antibiotic-refractory Lyme arthritis is associated with HLA-DR molecules that bind a Borrelia burgdorferi peptide. *J Exp Med.* 2006;203(4):961-971.

48. Wormser GP, Brisson D, Liveris D, et al. Borrelia burgdorferi genotype predicts the capacity for hematogenous dissemination during early Lyme disease. *J Infect Dis.* 2008;198(9):1358-1364.

49. Rudenko N, Golovchenko M, Grubhoffer L, Oliver JH, Jr. Borrelia carolinensis sp. nov., a new (14th) member of the Borrelia burgdorferi Sensu Lato complex from the southeastern region of the United States. *J Clin Microbiol.* 2009;47(1):134-141.

50. Rudenko N, Golovchenko M, Lin T, Gao L, Grubhoffer L, Oliver JH, Jr. Delineation of a new species of the Borrelia burgdorferi Sensu Lato Complex, Borrelia americana sp. nov. *J Clin Microbiol.* 2009;47(12):3875-3880.

51. Rudenko N, Golovchenko M, Mokracek A, et al. Detection of Borrelia bissettii in cardiac valve tissue of a patient with endocarditis and aortic valve stenosis in the Czech Republic. *J Clin Microbiol.* 2008;46(10):3540-3543.

52. Rudenko N, Golovchenko M, Ruzek D, Piskunova N, Mallatova N, Grubhoffer L. Molecular detection of Borrelia bissettii DNA in serum samples from patients in the Czech

Republic with suspected borreliosis. *FEMS Microbiol Lett.* 2009;292(2):274-281.

53. Jones SG, Coulter S, Conner W. Using administrative medical claims data to supplement state disease registry systems for reporting zoonotic infections. *J Am Med Inform Assoc.* 2012.

54. Enhancing Lyme Disease Surveillance by Using Administrative Claims Data, Tennessee, USA Available from http://wwwnc.cdc.gov/eid/article/21/9/15-0344_article Last accessed 8/2/15.

55. Wang P, Glowacki MN, Hoet AE, et al. Emergence of Ixodes scapularis and Borrelia burgdorferi, the Lyme disease vector and agent, in Ohio. *Frontiers in cellular and infection microbiology.* 2014;4:70.

56. Moutailler S, Valiente Moro C, Vaumourin E, et al. Co-infection of Ticks: The Rule Rather Than the Exception. *PLoS Negl Trop Dis.* 2016;10(3):e0004539.

57. Telford SR, 3rd, Wormser GP. Bartonella spp. transmission by ticks not established. *Emerg Infect Dis.* 2010;16(3):379-384.

58. Diuk-Wasser MA, Vannier E, Krause PJ. Coinfection by Ixodes Tick-Borne Pathogens: Ecological, Epidemiological, and Clinical Consequences. *Trends Parasitol.* 2015.

59. Hersh MH, Ostfeld RS, McHenry DJ, et al. Co-infection of blacklegged ticks with Babesia microti and Borrelia burgdorferi is higher than expected and acquired from small mammal hosts. *PLoS One.* 2014;9(6):e99348.

60. Krause PJ, Telford SR, 3rd, Spielman A, et al. Concurrent Lyme disease and babesiosis. Evidence for increased severity and duration of illness. *Jama.* 1996;275(21):1657-1660.

61. Curcio SR, Tria LP, Gucwa AL. Seroprevalence of Babesia microti in Individuals with Lyme Disease. *Vector Borne Zoonotic Dis.* 2016;16(12):737-743.

62. Tonnetti L, Thorp AM, Deisting B, et al. Babesia microti

seroprevalence in Minnesota blood donors. *Transfusion.* 2013;53(8):1698-1705.

63. Bullard JM, Ahsanuddin AN, Perry AM, et al. The first case of locally acquired tick-borne Babesia microti infection in Canada. *Can J Infect Dis Med Microbiol.* 2014;25(6):e87-89.

64. Telford SR, 3rd, Goethert HK, Molloy PJ, et al. Borrelia miyamotoi Disease: Neither Lyme Disease Nor Relapsing Fever. *Clin Lab Med.* 2015;35(4):867-882.

65. Molloy PJ, Telford Iii SR, Chowdri HR, et al. Borrelia miyamotoi Disease in the Northeastern United States: A Case Series. *Ann Intern Med.* 2015.

66. Binnicker MJ, Theel ES, Pritt BS. Lack of evidence for rapid transmission of Lyme disease following a tick bite. *Diagn Microbiol Infect Dis.* 2012;73(1):102-103.

67. New Cause for Lyme Disease Complicates Already Murky Diagnosis, By Melinda Wenner Moyer, February 16, 2016, in Scientific American. at http://www.scientificamerican.com/article/new-cause-for-lyme-disease-complicates-already-murky-diagnosis1/. Last accessed 2/20/16.

68. Logigian EL, Kaplan RF, Steere AC. Successful treatment of Lyme encephalopathy with intravenous ceftriaxone. *J Infect Dis.* 1999;180(2):377-383.

69. Cameron DJ, Johnson LB, Maloney EL. Evidence assessments and guideline recommendations in Lyme disease: the clinical management of known tick bites, erythema migrans rashes and persistent disease. *Expert Rev Anti Infect Ther.* 2014:1-33.

70. Wormser GP, Dattwyler RJ, Shapiro ED, et al. The clinical assessment, treatment, and prevention of lyme disease, human granulocytic anaplasmosis, and babesiosis: clinical practice guidelines by the Infectious Diseases Society of America. *Clin Infect Dis.* 2006;43(9):1089-1134.

71. Kanjwal K, Karabin B, Kanjwal Y, Grubb BP. Postural orthostatic tachycardia syndrome following Lyme disease. *Cardiol J.* 2011;18(1):63-66.

72. Fallon BA, Nields JA, Burrascano JJ, Liegner K, DelBene D, Liebowitz MR. The neuropsychiatric manifestations of Lyme borreliosis. *Psychiatr Q.* 1992;63(1):95-117.

73. Krupp LB, Hyman LG, Grimson R, et al. Study and treatment of post Lyme disease (STOP-LD): a randomized double masked clinical trial. *Neurology.* 2003;60(12):1923-1930.

74. Mygland A, Ljostad U, Fingerle V, Rupprecht T, Schmutzhard E, Steiner I. EFNS guidelines on the diagnosis and management of European Lyme neuroborreliosis. *European journal of neurology : the official journal of the European Federation of Neurological Societies.* 2010;17(1):8-16, e11-14.

75. Aucott JN. Posttreatment Lyme disease syndrome. *Infect Dis Clin North Am.* 2015;29(2):309-323.

76. Asch ES, Bujak DI, Weiss M, Peterson MG, Weinstein A. Lyme disease: an infectious and postinfectious syndrome. *J Rheumatol.* 1994;21(3):454-461.

77. Shadick NA, Phillips CB, Logigian EL, et al. The long-term clinical outcomes of Lyme disease. A population-based retrospective cohort study. *Ann Intern Med.* 1994;121(8):560-567.

78. Halperin JJ. Neuroborreliosis: central nervous system involvement. *Semin Neurol.* 1997;17(1):19-24.

79. Sathiamoorthi S, Smith WM. The eye and tick-borne disease in the United States. *Curr Opin Ophthalmol.* 2016;27(6):530-537.

80. Sudharshan S, Ganesh SK, Biswas J. Current approach in the diagnosis and management of posterior uveitis. *Indian J Ophthalmol.* 2010;58(1):29-43.

81. Agrawal RV, Murthy S, Sangwan V, Biswas J. Current approach in

diagnosis and management of anterior uveitis. *Indian J Ophthalmol.* 2010;58(1):11-19.

82. Pendse S, Bilyk JR, Lee MS. The ticking time bomb. *Surv Ophthalmol.* 2006;51(3):274-279.

83. LeWitt TM. Hemifacial Spasm From Lyme Disease: Antibiotic Treatment Points to the Cause. *Clin Neuropharmacol.* 2016.

84. Basile RC, Yoshinari NH, Mantovani E, Bonoldi VN, Macoris DD, Queiroz-Neto A. Brazilian borreliosis with special emphasis on humans and horses. *Braz J Microbiol.* 2016.

85. Shih CM, Spielman A. Accelerated transmission of Lyme disease spirochetes by partially fed vector ticks. *J Clin Microbiol.* 1993;31(11):2878-2881.

86. White M, Meenan K, Patel T, Jaworek A, Sataloff RT. Laboratory Evaluation of Vocal Fold Paralysis and Paresis. *J Voice.* 2016.

87. Schroeter V, Belz GG, Blenk H. Paralysis of recurrent laryngeal nerve in Lyme disease. *Lancet.* 1988;2(8622):1245.

88. Martzolff L, Bouhala M, Dukic R, et al. [Recurrent nerve palsy due to Lyme disease: report of two cases]. *Rev Med Interne.* 2010;31(3):229-231.

89. Puri BK, Shah M, Julu PO, Kingston MC, Monro JA. The association of lyme disease with loss of sexual libido and the role of urinary bladder detrusor dysfunction. *International neurourology journal.* 2014;18(2):95-97.

90. Nowakowski J, McKenna D, Nadelman RB, et al. Failure of treatment with cephalexin for Lyme disease. *Arch Fam Med.* 2000;9(6):563-567.

91. Patel LD, Schachne JS. Lyme Carditis: A Case Involving the Conduction System and Mitral Valve. *R I Med J (2013).* 2017;100(2):17-20.

92. Fishe JN, Marchese RF, Callahan JM. Lyme Myocarditis Presenting as Chest Pain in an Adolescent Girl. *Pediatr Emerg Care.* 2016.

93. Robinson J, Hartling L, Vandermeer B, Crumley E, Klassen TP. Intravenous immunoglobulin for presumed viral myocarditis in children and adults. *Cochrane Database Syst Rev.* 2005(1):CD004370.

94. Muehlenbachs A, Bollweg BC, Schulz TJ, et al. Cardiac Tropism of Borrelia burgdorferi: An Autopsy Study of Sudden Cardiac Death Associated with Lyme Carditis. *Am J Pathol.* 2016.

95. Blackwell WA. Early Disseminated Lyme Disease. *Mayo Clin Proc.* 2017;92(4):687-688.

96. Gone in a Heartbeat: A Physician's Search for True Healing by Neil Spector at My Book. Last accessed 3/23/17.

97. Neil Spector, MD, Show 996: Mystery and Lyme Disease Misdiagnosis (Archive) on 2015 at https://www.peoplespharmacy.com/2016/05/19/show-996-mystery-and-lyme-disease-misdiagnosis/. Last accessed 5/1/17.

98. Yoon EC, Vail E, Kleinman G, et al. Lyme disease: a case report of a 17-year-old male with fatal Lyme carditis. *Cardiovasc Pathol.* 2015;24(5):317-321.

99. Patel R, Larnard J, Poowanawittayakom N, Glew R. 1800: Atypical Lyme Meningitis with Parkinson Disease-Like Manifestations. *Crit Care Med.* 2016;44(12 Suppl 1):525.

100. Mitra K, Gangopadhaya PK, Das SK. Parkinsonism plus syndrome--a review. *Neurol India.* 2003;51(2):183-188.

101. Williams DR, Litvan I. Parkinsonian syndromes. *Continuum (Minneap Minn).* 2013;19(5 Movement Disorders):1189-1212.

102. Pische G, Koob M, Wirth T, et al. Subacute parkinsonism as a complication of Lyme disease. *J Neurol.* 2017.

103. Seifert KD, Wiener JI. The impact of DaTscan on the diagnosis

and management of movement disorders: A retrospective study. *Am J Neurodegener Dis.* 2013;2(1):29-34.

104. Garkowski A, Zajkowska J, Zajkowska A, et al. Cerebrovascular Manifestations of Lyme Neuroborreliosis-A Systematic Review of Published Cases. *Front Neurol.* 2017;8:146.

105. Almoussa M, Goertzen A, Fauser B, Zimmermann CW. Stroke as an Unusual First Presentation of Lyme Disease. *Case Rep Neurol Med.* 2015;2015:389081.

106. Kris Kristofferson: An Outlaw at 80. by Neil Strauss in Rolling Stone at http://www.rollingstone.com/music/features/kris-kristofferson-an-outlaw-at-80-20160606. Last accessed 6/12/16.

107. He beat leukemia. But then, mysteriously, things got really bad. by Sandra G. Boodman at https://www.washingtonpost.com/national/health-science/he-beat-leukemia-but-then-mysteriously-things-got-really-bad/2016/06/06/1178d9f0-0564-11e6-a12f-ea5aed7958dc_story.html. Last accessed 6/12/16.

108. Topakian R, Artemian H, Metschitzer B, Lugmayr H, Kuhr T, Pischinger B. Dramatic response to a 3-week course of ceftriaxone in late neuroborreliosis mimicking atypical dementia and normal pressure hydrocephalus. *J Neurol Sci.* 2016;366:146-148.

109. Lynch MC, Milchak MA, Parnes H, Ioffreda MD. Tick Bite Alopecia: A Report and Review. *Am J Dermatopathol.* 2016;38(11):e150-e153.

110. Ross MS, Friede H. Alopecia due to tick bite. *AMA Arch Derm.* 1955;71(4):524-525.

111. Heyl T. Tick bite alopecia. *Clin Exp Dermatol.* 1982;7(5):537-542.

112. Krinsky WL. Dermatoses associated with the bites of mites and ticks (Arthropoda: Acari). *Int J Dermatol.* 1983;22(2):75-91.

113. Raoult D, Lakos A, Fenollar F, Beytout J, Brouqui P, Fournier PE.

Spotless rickettsiosis caused by Rickettsia slovaca and associated with Dermacentor ticks. *Clin Infect Dis.* 2002;34(10):1331-1336.

114.Cimperman J, Maraspin V, Lotric-Furlan S, Ruzic-Sabljic E, Avsic-Zupanc T, Strle F. Diffuse reversible alopecia in patients with Lyme meningitis and tick-borne encephalitis. *Wien Klin Wochenschr.* 1999;111(22-23):976-977.

115.Moghadam-Kia S, Franks AG, Jr. Autoimmune disease and hair loss. *Dermatol Clin.* 2013;31(1):75-91.

116.Wang TJ, Liang MH, Sangha O, et al. Coexposure to Borrelia burgdorferi and Babesia microti does not worsen the long-term outcome of lyme disease. *Clin Infect Dis.* 2000;31(5):1149-1154.

117.Golightly LM, Hirschhorn LR, Weller PF. Fever and headache in a splenectomized woman. *Rev Infect Dis.* 1989;11(4):629-637.

118.Marcus LC, Steere AC, Duray PH, Anderson AE, Mahoney EB. Fatal pancarditis in a patient with coexistent Lyme disease and babesiosis. Demonstration of spirochetes in the myocardium. *Ann Intern Med.* 1985;103(3):374-376.

119.Krause PJ, McKay K, Thompson CA, et al. Disease-specific diagnosis of coinfecting tickborne zoonoses: babesiosis, human granulocytic ehrlichiosis, and Lyme disease. *Clin Infect Dis.* 2002;34(9):1184-1191.

120.Krause PJ, Feder HM, Jr. Lyme disease and babesiosis. *Adv Pediatr Infect Dis.* 1994;9:183-209.

121.Steere AC, McHugh G, Suarez C, Hoitt J, Damle N, Sikand VK. Prospective study of coinfection in patients with erythema migrans. *Clin Infect Dis.* 2003;36(8):1078-1081.

122.Former N.J. First Lady Jean Byrne dies at 88 from nj.com August 11, 2015 at http://www.nj.com/mercer/index.ssf/2015/08/jean_byrne_former_nj_first_lady_dies_at_88.html. Last accessed 9/25/17.

123. Bechtold KT, Rebman AW, Crowder LA, Johnson-Greene D, Aucott JN. Standardized Symptom Measurement of Individuals with Early Lyme Disease Over Time. *Arch Clin Neuropsychol.* 2017;32(2):129-141.

124. Klempner MS. Controlled trials of antibiotic treatment in patients with post-treatment chronic Lyme disease. *Vector Borne Zoonotic Dis.* 2002;2(4):255-263.

125. Berende A, ter Hofstede HJ, Vos FJ, et al. Randomized Trial of Longer-Term Therapy for Symptoms Attributed to Lyme Disease. *N Engl J Med.* 2016;374(13):1209-1220.

126. Cameron D. Severity of Lyme disease with persistent symptoms. Insights from a double-blind placebo-controlled clinical trial. *Minerva Med.* 2008;99(5):489-496.

127. Melia MT, Lantos PM, Auwaerter PG. Lyme Disease: Authentic Imitator or Wishful Imitation? *JAMA neurology.* 2014.

128. Wormser GP. Longer-Term Therapy for Symptoms Attributed to Lyme Disease. *N Engl J Med.* 2016;375(10):997.

129. Wormser GP, Sudhindra P, Lopez E, et al. Fatigue in patients with erythema migrans. *Diagn Microbiol Infect Dis.* 2016.

130. Aucott JN, Soloski MJ, Rebman AW, et al. CCL19 as a Chemokine Risk Factor for Post-Treatment Lyme Disease Syndrome: A Prospective Clinical Cohort Study. *Clin Vaccine Immunol.* 2016.

131. Weitzner E, Visintainer P, Wormser GP. Comparison of males versus females with culture-confirmed early Lyme disease at presentation and at 11-20 years after diagnosis. *Diagn Microbiol Infect Dis.* 2016.

132. Zhang X, Meltzer MI, Pena CA, Hopkins AB, Wroth L, Fix AD. Economic impact of Lyme disease. *Emerg Infect Dis.* 2006;12(4):653-660.

133. Wills AB, Spaulding AB, Adjemian J, et al. Long-term follow-up of

patients with Lyme disease: Longitudinal analysis of clinical and quality of life measures. *Clin Infect Dis.* 2016.

134. ClinicalTrials.Gov. Evaluation, Treatment, and Follow-up of Patients With Lyme Disease at https://clinicaltrials.gov/ct2/show/NCT00028080. Last accessed 4/20/16.

135. Dersch R, Sarnes AA, Maul M, et al. Quality of life, fatigue, depression and cognitive impairment in Lyme neuroborreliosis. *J Neurol.* 2015.

136. Silverman S, Dukes EM, Johnston SS, Brandenburg NA, Sadosky A, Huse DM. The economic burden of fibromyalgia: comparative analysis with rheumatoid arthritis. *Curr Med Res Opin.* 2009;25(4):829-840.

137. Clarke AE, Esdaile JM, Bloch DA, Lacaille D, Danoff DS, Fries JF. A Canadian study of the total medical costs for patients with systemic lupus erythematosus and the predictors of costs. *Arthritis Rheum.* 1993;36(11):1548-1559.

138. Kuehn BM. CDC estimates 300,000 US cases of Lyme disease annually. *Jama.* 2013;310(11):1110.

139. Adrion ER, Aucott J, Lemke KW, Weiner JP. Health care costs, utilization and patterns of care following Lyme disease. *PLoS One.* 2015;10(2):e0116767.

140. Lyme Disease Costs Up to $1.3 Billion Per Year to Treat, Study Finds, Johns Hopkins Bloomberg School of Publc Health News, February 5,2015 from http://www.jhsph.edu/news/news-releases/2015/lyme-disease-costs-more-than-one-billion-dollars-per-year-to-treat-study-finds.html. Last accessed 4/5/17.

141. Lantos PM, Branda JA, Boggan JC, et al. Poor positive predictive value of Lyme disease serologic testing in an area of low disease incidence. *Clin Infect Dis.* 2015.

142. Connally NP, Hinckley AF, Feldman KA, et al. Testing practices

and volume of non-Lyme tickborne diseases in the United States. *Ticks Tick Borne Dis.* 2016;7(1):193-198.

143. Gasmi S, Ogden NH, Leighton PA, Lindsay LR, Thivierge K. Analysis of the human population bitten by Ixodes scapularis ticks in Quebec, Canada: Increasing risk of Lyme disease. *Ticks Tick Borne Dis.* 2016.

144. Dibernardo A, Cote T, Ogden NH, Lindsay LR. The prevalence of Borrelia miyamotoi infection, and co-infections with other Borrelia spp. in Ixodes scapularis ticks collected in Canada. *Parasit Vectors.* 2014;7:183.

145. Wilson IG. Inhibition and facilitation of nucleic acid amplification. *Appl Environ Microbiol.* 1997;63(10):3741-3751.

146. Krause PJ, Lepore T, Sikand VK, et al. Atovaquone and azithromycin for the treatment of babesiosis. *N Engl J Med.* 2000;343(20):1454-1458.

147. Perronne C, Lacout A, Marcy PY, El Hajjam M. Errancy on Lyme Diagnosis. *Am J Med.* 2017;130(5):e219.

148. Cameron DJ. Consequences of treatment delay in Lyme disease. *J Eval Clin Pract.* 2007;13(3):470-472.

149. Pavletic AJ, Marques AR. Early Disseminated Lyme Disease Causing False Positive Serology for Primary Epstein-Barr Virus Infection - Report of 2 Cases. *Clin Infect Dis.* 2017.

150. Krause PJ, Narasimhan S, Wormser GP, et al. Human Borrelia miyamotoi infection in the United States. *N Engl J Med.* 2013;368(3):291-293.

151. Chowdri HR, Gugliotta JL, Berardi VP, et al. Borrelia miyamotoi infection presenting as human granulocytic anaplasmosis: a case report. *Ann Intern Med.* 2013;159(1):21-27.

152. Padgett K, Bonilla D, Kjemtrup A, et al. Large Scale Spatial Risk and Comparative Prevalence of Borrelia miyamotoi and Borrelia

burgdorferi Sensu Lato in Ixodes pacificus. *PLoS One.* 2014;9(10):e110853.

153. Dworkin MS, Schwan TG, Anderson DE, Jr., Borchardt SM. Tick-borne relapsing fever. *Infect Dis Clin North Am.* 2008;22(3):449-468, viii.

154. Gugliotta JL, Goethert HK, Berardi VP, Telford SR, 3rd. Meningoencephalitis from Borrelia miyamotoi in an immunocompromised patient. *N Engl J Med.* 2013;368(3):240-245.

155. Hovius JW, de Wever B, Sohne M, et al. A case of meningoencephalitis by the relapsing fever spirochaete Borrelia miyamotoi in Europe. *Lancet.* 2013;382(9892):658.

156. Mantilla-Florez YF, Faccini-Martinez AA, Perez-Diaz CE. American woman with early Lyme borreliosis diagnosed in a Colombian hospital. *Travel Med Infect Dis.* 2017.

157. Sudhindra P, Wang G, Schriefer ME, et al. Insights into Borrelia miyamotoi infection from an untreated case demonstrating relapsing fever, monocytosis and a positive C6 Lyme serology. *Diagn Microbiol Infect Dis.* 2016;86(1):93-96.

158. Neves N, Silva-Pinto A, Rocha H, et al. Plasmodium spp. and Borrelia burgdorferi co-infection associated with antiphospholipid syndrome in a returned traveler: a case report. *Clin Case Rep.* 2017;5(4):471-476.

159. Cooper L, Branagan-Harris M, Tuson R, Nduka C. Lyme disease and Bell's palsy: an epidemiological study of diagnosis and risk in England. *Br J Gen Pract.* 2017.

160. Homer MJ, Aguilar-Delfin I, Telford SR, 3rd, Krause PJ, Persing DH. Babesiosis. *Clin Microbiol Rev.* 2000;13(3):451-469.

161. Ramsey AH, Belongia EA, Chyou PH, Davis JP. Appropriateness of Lyme disease serologic testing. *Ann Fam Med.* 2004;2(4):341-344.

162. Mold JW, Holtzclaw BJ, McCarthy L. Night sweats: a systematic review of the literature. *J Am Board Fam Med.* 2012;25(6):878-893.

163. Thaisetthawatkul P, Logigian EL. Peripheral nervous system manifestations of lyme borreliosis. *J Clin Neuromuscul Dis.* 2002;3(4):165-171.

164. Strle F, Ruzic E, Cimperman J. Erythema migrans: comparison of treatment with azithromycin, doxycycline and phenoxymethylpenicillin. *J Antimicrob Chemother.* 1992;30(4):543-550.

165. Time to Become Familiar With Babesiosis? by Paul G. Auwaerter July 1, 2015 at http://www.medscape.com/viewarticle/846942. Last accessed 2/27/17.

166. Zaiem F, Alkawam H, Lee S, Fabisevich M. Severe Symptomatic Babesiosis Co-infection with Lyme Disease. *QJM.* 2015.

167. Oleson CV, Sivalingam JJ, O'Neill BJ, Staas WE, Jr. Transverse myelitis secondary to coexistent Lyme disease and babesiosis. *J Spinal Cord Med.* 2003;26(2):168-171.

168. Brunner M, Sigal LH. Use of serum immune complexes in a new test that accurately confirms early Lyme disease and active infection with Borrelia burgdorferi. *J Clin Microbiol.* 2001;39(9):3213-3221.

169. Schutzer SE, Coyle PK, Belman AL, Golightly MG, Drulle J. Sequestration of antibody to Borrelia burgdorferi in immune complexes in seronegative Lyme disease. *Lancet.* 1990;335(8685):312-315.

170. Singh SK, Girschick HJ. Lyme borreliosis: from infection to autoimmunity. *Clin Microbiol Infect.* 2004;10(7):598-614.

171. Dattwyler RJ, Volkman DJ, Luft BJ, Halperin JJ, Thomas J, Golightly MG. Seronegative Lyme disease. Dissociation of specific T- and B-lymphocyte responses to Borrelia burgdorferi. *N Engl J Med.* 1988;319(22):1441-1446.

172. Steere AC. Seronegative Lyme disease. *Jama.* 1993;270(11):1369.

173. Dressler F, Yoshinari NH, Steere AC. The T-cell proliferative assay in the diagnosis of Lyme disease. *Ann Intern Med.* 1991;115(7):533-539.

174. Schutzer SE, Coyle PK, Reid P, Holland B. Borrelia burgdorferi-specific immune complexes in acute Lyme disease. *Jama.* 1999;282(20):1942-1946.

175. Brunner M. New method for detection of Borrelia burgdorferi antigen complexed to antibody in seronegative Lyme disease. *J Immunol Methods.* 2001;249(1-2):185-190.

176. Kantor FS. Disarming Lyme disease. *Sci Am.* 1994;271(3):34-39.

177. Ang CW, Notermans DW, Hommes M, Simoons-Smit AM, Herremans T. Large differences between test strategies for the detection of anti-Borrelia antibodies are revealed by comparing eight ELISAs and five immunoblots. *Eur J Clin Microbiol Infect Dis.* 2011.

178. Fallon BA, Kochevar JM, Gaito A, Nields JA. The underdiagnosis of neuropsychiatric Lyme disease in children and adults. *Psychiatr Clin North Am.* 1998;21(3):693-703, viii.

179. Pachner AR. Borrelia burgdorferi in the nervous system: the new "great imitator". *Ann N Y Acad Sci.* 1988;539:56-64.

180. Miner JJ, Aw Yeang HX, Fox JM, et al. Chikungunya viral arthritis in the United States: a mimic of seronegative rheumatoid arthritis. *Arthritis & rheumatology.* 2015;67(5):1214-1220.

181. Eugene Shapiro, MD, on suspected Lyme disease Meeting News Coverage from the Pediatric Academic Societies Annual Meeting in Healio Infectious Diseases in Children on May 12, 2014 at http://www.healio.com/pediatrics/emerging-diseases/news/online/%7Bb39f5e7e-7aba-434a-8f5d-7ce416bdef73%7D/eugene-shapiro-md-on-suspected-lyme-disease. Last accessed 4/26/17.

182. Unigwe C, Rowett M, Udo I. Reflections on the management of

medically unexplained symptoms. *The psychiatric bulletin.* 2014;38(5):252.

183. Isaac ML, Paauw DS. Medically unexplained symptoms. *The Medical clinics of North America.* 2014;98(3):663-672.

184. Lebowitz MS, Ahn WK. Effects of biological explanations for mental disorders on clinicians' empathy. *Proc Natl Acad Sci U S A.* 2014;111(50):17786-17790.

185. Bradley LA, Wohlreich MM, Wang F, et al. Pain response profile of patients with fibromyalgia treated with duloxetine. *Clin J Pain.* 2010;26(6):498-504.

186. Vitton O, Gendreau M, Gendreau J, Kranzler J, Rao SG. A double-blind placebo-controlled trial of milnacipran in the treatment of fibromyalgia. *Hum Psychopharmacol.* 2004;19 Suppl 1:S27-35.

187. Straube S, Derry S, Moore RA, McQuay HJ. Pregabalin in fibromyalgia: meta-analysis of efficacy and safety from company clinical trial reports. *Rheumatology (Oxford).* 2010;49(4):706-715.

188. Cassisi G, Sarzi-Puttini P, Alciati A, et al. Symptoms and signs in fibromyalgia syndrome. *Reumatismo.* 2008;60 Suppl 1:15-24.

189. Wolfe F, Smythe HA, Yunus MB, et al. The American College of Rheumatology 1990 Criteria for the Classification of Fibromyalgia. Report of the Multicenter Criteria Committee. *Arthritis Rheum.* 1990;33(2):160-172.

190. Steere AC, Snydman D, Murray P, et al. Historical perspective of Lyme disease. *Zentralbl Bakteriol Mikrobiol Hyg [A].* 1986;263(1-2):3-6.

191. Milewski MD, Cruz AI, Jr., Miller CP, Peterson AT, Smith BG. Lyme arthritis in children presenting with joint effusions. *J Bone Joint Surg Am.* 2011;93(3):252-260.

192. Jennings F, Lambert E, Fredericson M. Rheumatic diseases presenting as sports-related injuries. *Sports Med.* 2008;38(11):917-930.

193. Sigal LH. Summary of the first 100 patients seen at a Lyme disease referral center. *Am J Med.* 1990;88(6):577-581.

194. Wormser GP, Dattwyler RJ, Shapiro ED, Halperin JJ, Steere AC, Klempner MS, Krause PJ, Bakken JS, Strle F, Stanek G, Bockenstedt L, Fish D, Dumler JS, Nadelman RB from The Clinical Assessment, Treatment, and Prevention of Lyme Disease, Human Granulocytic Anaplasmosis, and Babesiosis: Clinical Practice Guidelines by the Infectious Diseases Society of America at https://www.google.com/url?sa=t&rct=j&q=&esrc=s&source=web&cd=4&cad=rja&uact=8&ved=0ahUKEwiIutDHtubKAhWCHD4KHdeaCDAQFggqMAM&url=http%3A%2F%2Fcid.oxfordjournals.org%2Fcontent%2F43%2F9%2F1089.full.pdf%2Bhtml&usg=AFQjCNG-0DoVRahmPc-MIgsGuYF8vlWDHw&sig2=mYgQYHhlifKomistPChX6A. Last accessed 2/7/16.

195. Cameron DJ, Johnson LB, Maloney EL. Evidence assessments and guideline recommendations in Lyme disease: the clinical management of known tick bites, erythema migrans rashes and persistent disease from Expert Review of Anti-infective Therapy 2014 at http://www.tandfonline.com/doi/full/10.1586/14787210.2014.940900. Last accessed 1/3/16.

196. Harvey WT, Salvato P. 'Lyme disease': ancient engine of an unrecognized borreliosis pandemic? *Med Hypotheses.* 2003;60(5):742-759.

197. Butler AD, Sedghi T, Petrini JR, Ahmadi R. Tick-borne disease preventive practices and perceptions in an endemic area. *Ticks Tick Borne Dis.* 2015.

198. Morens DM, Folkers GK, Fauci AS. What is a pandemic? *J Infect Dis.* 2009;200(7):1018-1021.

199. Sanchez E, Vannier E, Wormser GP, Hu LT. Diagnosis, Treatment, and Prevention of Lyme Disease, Human Granulocytic Anaplasmosis, and Babesiosis: A Review. *Jama.* 2016;315(16):1767-1777.

200. Cairns V, Godwin J. Post-Lyme borreliosis syndrome: a meta-analysis of reported symptoms. *Int J Epidemiol.* 2005;34(6):1340-1345.

201. Borgermans L, Perronne C, Balicer R, Polasek O, Obsomer V. Lyme disease: time for a new approach? *BMJ.* 2015;351:h6520.

202. Borgermans L, Goderis G, Vandevoorde J, Devroey D. Relevance of chronic lyme disease to family medicine as a complex multidimensional chronic disease construct: a systematic review. *Int J Family Med.* 2014;2014:138016.

203. Shapiro ED, Baker PJ, Wormser GP. False and Misleading Information about Lyme Disease. *Am J Med.* 2017.

204. "Doctors and Patients Team Up for Better Health", Pittsburgh Post-Gazette by David Templeton on 10/27/15 at http://www.post-gazette.com/news/health/2015/10/27/Doctors-and-patients-team-up-for-better-health/stories/201510270008. Last accessed 3/24/17.

205. Shared Decision Making Philosophy, from the Mayo Clinic Shared Decision Making National Resource Center at http://shareddecisions.mayoclinic.org/decision-aid-information/decision-aids-for-chronic-disease/. Last accessed 3/24/17.

206. Lantos PM. Chronic Lyme Disease. *Infect Dis Clin North Am.* 2015;29(2):325-340.

207. What CDC is Doing . CDC in action: What CDC is doing to help at https://www.cdc.gov/zika/about/whatcdcisdoing.html. Last accessed 5/7/17.

208. This Mosquito Likes Us Too Much For Our Own Good, by Jason Beaubien, February 12, 2016 at http://www.npr.org/sections/goatsandsoda/2016/02/10/466268138/this-mosquito-likes-us-too-much-for-our-own-good Last accessed 2/13/16.

209. Mission, Role and Pledge from the Centers for Disease Control and Prevention CDC24/7 Saving Lives, Protecting People at https://

www.cdc.gov/about/organization/mission.htm. Last accessed 9/24/17.

210. Wormser GP, McKenna D, Nowakowski J. Management approaches for suspected and established Lyme disease used at the Lyme disease diagnostic center. *Wien Klin Wochenschr.* 2016.

211. Wormser GP, Weitzner E, McKenna D, et al. Long-term Assessment of Health-Related Quality of Life in Patients With Culture-Confirmed Early Lyme Disease. *Clin Infect Dis.* 2015.

212. Wormser GP, Weitzner E, McKenna D, Nadelman RB, Scavarda C, Nowakowski J. Long-term assessment of fatigue in patients with culture-confirmed Lyme disease. *Am J Med.* 2015;128(2):181-184.

213. Wormser GP, Weitzner E, McKenna D, et al. Long-Term Assessment of Fibromyalgia in Patients with Culture-Confirmed Lyme Disease. *Arthritis & rheumatology.* 2014.

214. Auwaerter PG. Life After Lyme Disease. *Clin Infect Dis.* 2015.

215. The GRADE Approach Video from the American Thoracic Society Published on Apr 16, 2008 at https://www.youtube.com/watch?v=x6MlqC7157E&feature=related. Last accessed 9/25/17.

216. Evidence assessments and guideline recommendations in Lyme disease: the clinical management of known tick bites, erythema migrans rashes and persistent disease. National Guideline Clearinghouse. Agency for Health Care Research and Quality. Available from: http://www.guideline.gov/content.aspx?id=49320. Last accessed 10/11/15.

217. http://www.ilads.org/. last accessed 5/8/16.

218. Altmetric Who's talking about your research? at https://www.altmetric.com/. Last accessed 5/8/16.

219. Macauda MM, Erickson P, Miller J, Mann P, Closter L, Krause PJ. Long-Term Lyme Disease Antibiotic Therapy Beliefs Among New England Residents. *Vector borne and zoonotic diseases.* 2011.

220. Tseng YJ, Cami A, Goldmann DA, DeMaria A, Jr., Mandl KD. Incidence and Patterns of Extended-Course Antibiotic Therapy in Patients Evaluated for Lyme Disease. *Clin Infect Dis.* 2015.

221. Zhao H, Bao FF, Liu A. Safety, immunogenicity, and efficacy of Borrelia burgdorferi outer surface protein A (OspA) vaccine: A meta-analysis. *J Infect Dev Ctries.* 2017;11(1):1-9.

222. FDA Package Insert - LYMErix™. Last accessed 3/5/12; http://www.fda.gov/ohrms/DOCKETS/ac/01/briefing/3680b2_03.pdf.

223. Steere AC, Sikand VK, Meurice F, et al. Vaccination against Lyme disease with recombinant Borrelia burgdorferi outer-surface lipoprotein A with adjuvant. Lyme Disease Vaccine Study Group. *N Engl J Med.* 1998;339(4):209-215.

224. Lyme disease vaccine, Centers for Disease Control and Prevention, Available from: http://www.cdc.gov/lyme/prev/vaccine.html. Last accessed 10/11/15.

225. Lyme Disease Treatment Would Prevent Infection, Researchers Say, by Maggie Fox at NBCNews.com Available from: http://www.nbcnews.com/health/health-news/lyme-disease-treatment-would-prevent-infection-researchers-say-n441946. Last accessed 10/11/15.

226. Oda R, Kutsuna S, Sekikawa Y, et al. The first case of imported Borrelia miyamotoi disease concurrent with Lyme disease. *J Infect Chemother.* 2017.

227. Schwan TG, Schrumpf ME, Hinnebusch BJ, Anderson DE, Jr., Konkel ME. GlpQ: an antigen for serological discrimination between relapsing fever and Lyme borreliosis. *J Clin Microbiol.* 1996;34(10):2483-2492.

228. Cochrane at http://www.cochrane.org/. Last accessed 9/24/17.

229. Cadavid D, Auwaerter PG, Rumbaugh J, Gelderblom H. Antibiotics for the neurological complications of Lyme disease. *Cochrane Database Syst Rev.* 2016;12:CD006978.

230. Applegren ND, Kraus CK. Lyme Disease: Emergency Department Considerations. *J Emerg Med.* 2017.

231. Feng J, Zhang S, Shi W, Zhang Y. Activity of Sulfa Drugs and Their Combinations against Stationary Phase B. burgdorferi In Vitro. *Antibiotics (Basel).* 2017;6(1).

232. De l'Etoile-Morel S, Feteih A, Hogan CA, Vinh D, Thanassoulis G. A Case of Reversible Complete Heart Block. *Am J Med.* 2017.

233. Fuster LS, Gul EE, Baranchuk A. Electrocardiographic progression of acute Lyme disease. *Am J Emerg Med.* 2017.

234. Jowett N, Gaudin RA, Banks CA, Hadlock TA. Steroid use in Lyme disease-associated facial palsy is associated with worse long-term outcomes. *Laryngoscope.* 2016.

235. Dattwyler RJ, Halperin JJ, Volkman DJ, Luft BJ. Treatment of late Lyme borreliosis--randomised comparison of ceftriaxone and penicillin. *Lancet.* 1988;1(8596):1191-1194.

236. Steere AC, Green J, Schoen RT, et al. Successful parenteral penicillin therapy of established Lyme arthritis. *N Engl J Med.* 1985;312(14):869-874.

237. Straubinger RK, Straubinger AF, Summers BA, Jacobson RH. Status of Borrelia burgdorferi infection after antibiotic treatment and the effects of corticosteroids: An experimental study. *J Infect Dis.* 2000;181(3):1069-1081.

238. Straubinger RK, Straubinger AF, Summers BA, Jacobson RH, Erb HN. Clinical manifestations, pathogenesis, and effect of antibiotic treatment on Lyme borreliosis in dogs. *Wien Klin Wochenschr.* 1998;110(24):874-881.

239. Ogrinc K, Lusa L, Lotric-Furlan S, et al. Course and Outcome of Early European Lyme Neuroborreliosis (Bannwarth's Syndrome) - Clinical and Laboratory Findings. *Clin Infect Dis.* 2016.

240. Steere AC, Hutchinson GJ, Rahn DW, et al. Treatment of the early manifestations of Lyme disease. *Ann Intern Med.* 1983;99(1):22-26.

241. Fallon BA, Schwartzberg M, Bransfield R, et al. Late-stage neuropsychiatric Lyme borreliosis. Differential diagnosis and treatment. *Psychosomatics.* 1995;36(3):295-300.

242. Wormser GP, Liveris D, Nowakowski J, et al. Association of specific subtypes of Borrelia burgdorferi with hematogenous dissemination in early Lyme disease. *J Infect Dis.* 1999;180(3):720-725.

243. Jones KL, Glickstein LJ, Damle N, Sikand VK, McHugh G, Steere AC. Borrelia burgdorferi genetic markers and disseminated disease in patients with early Lyme disease. *J Clin Microbiol.* 2006;44(12):4407-4413.

244. Seinost G, Dykhuizen DE, Dattwyler RJ, et al. Four clones of Borrelia burgdorferi sensu stricto cause invasive infection in humans. *Infect Immun.* 1999;67(7):3518-3524.

245. Seemanapalli SV, Xu Q, McShan K, Liang FT. Outer surface protein C is a dissemination-facilitating factor of Borrelia burgdorferi during mammalian infection. *PloS one.* 2010;5(12):e15830.

246. Strle K, Drouin EE, Shen S, et al. Borrelia burgdorferi stimulates macrophages to secrete higher levels of cytokines and chemokines than Borrelia afzelii or Borrelia garinii. *The Journal of infectious diseases.* 2009;200(12):1936-1943.

247. Widhe M, Grusell M, Ekerfelt C, Vrethem M, Forsberg P, Ernerudh J. Cytokines in Lyme borreliosis: lack of early tumour necrosis factor-alpha and transforming growth factor-beta1 responses are associated with chronic neuroborreliosis. *Immunology.* 2002;107(1):46-55.

248. Wang G, Ojaimi C, Wu H, et al. Disease severity in a murine model of lyme borreliosis is associated with the genotype of the infecting Borrelia burgdorferi sensu stricto strain. *J Infect Dis.* 2002;186(6):782-791.

249. Walter KS, Carpi G, Evans BR, Caccone A, Diuk-Wasser MA. Vectors as Epidemiological Sentinels: Patterns of Within-Tick Borrelia burgdorferi Diversity. *PLoS Pathog.* 2016;12(7):e1005759.

250. "Stephen Jay Gould" (Interview by Michael Krasny). Mother Jones (Jan.-Feb. 1997): 60-63. (c)1997, Mother Jones at https://prelectur.stanford.edu/lecturers/gould/excerpts/index.html. Last accessed 9/24/17.

251. Feng J, Weitner M, Shi W, Zhang S, Sullivan D, Zhang Y. Identification of Additional Anti-Persister Activity against Borrelia burgdorferi from an FDA Drug Library. *Antibiotics (Basel).* 2015;4(3):397-410.

252. Feng J, Shi W, Zhang S, Sullivan D, Auwaerter PG, Zhang Y. A Drug Combination Screen Identifies Drugs Active against Amoxicillin-Induced Round Bodies of In Vitro Borrelia burgdorferi Persisters from an FDA Drug Library. *Front Microbiol.* 2016;7:743.

253. Feng J, Auwaerter PG, Zhang Y. Drug combinations against Borrelia burgdorferi persisters in vitro: eradication achieved by using daptomycin, cefoperazone and doxycycline. *PLoS One.* 2015;10(3):e0117207.

254. Miklossy J, Kasas S, Zurn AD, McCall S, Yu S, McGeer PL. Persisting atypical and cystic forms of Borrelia burgdorferi and local inflammation in Lyme neuroborreliosis. *J Neuroinflammation.* 2008;5:40.

255. Lantos PM, Auwaerter PG, Wormser GP. A systematic review of Borrelia burgdorferi morphologic variants does not support a role in chronic Lyme disease. *Clin Infect Dis.* 2014;58(5):663-671.

256. Arvikar SL, Crowley JT, Sulka KB, Steere AC. Autoimmune Arthritides, Rheumatoid Arthritis, Psoriatic Arthritis, or Peripheral Spondyloarthropathy, Following Lyme Disease. *Arthritis & rheumatology.* 2016.

257. Lau CS, Chamberlain RS. Probiotics are effective at preventing

Clostridium difficile-associated diarrhea: a systematic review and meta-analysis. *International Journal of General Medicine.* 2016;9:27-37.

258.Eppes SC, Childs JA. Comparative study of cefuroxime axetil versus amoxicillin in children with early Lyme disease. *Pediatrics.* 2002;109(6):1173-1177.

259.Holzbauer SM, Kemperman MM, Lynfield R. Death due to community-associated Clostridium difficile in a woman receiving prolonged antibiotic therapy for suspected lyme disease. *Clin Infect Dis.* 2010;51(3):369-370.

260.Nadelman RB, Arlin Z, Wormser GP. Life-threatening complications of empiric ceftriaxone therapy for 'seronegative Lyme disease'. *South Med J.* 1991;84(10):1263-1265.

261.Cammarota G, Masucci L, Ianiro G, et al. Randomised clinical trial: faecal microbiota transplantation by colonoscopy vs. vancomycin for the treatment of recurrent Clostridium difficile infection. *Aliment Pharmacol Ther.* 2015;41(9):835-843.

262.Garakani A, Mitton AG. New-onset panic, depression with suicidal thoughts, and somatic symptoms in a patient with a history of lyme disease. *Case Rep Psychiatry.* 2015;2015:457947.

263.What a year. from the Massachusetts Society for Medical Research newsletter. June 2016. at http://www.whatayear.org/06_16.php. Last accessed 9/25/17.

264.MassBiologics. at https://www.umassmed.edu/massbiologics/. Last accessed 9/25/17.

265.What you need to know about Borrelia miyamotoi. Centers for Disease Control and Prevention (CDC) Available from: http://www.cdc.gov/ticks/miyamotoi.html. Last accessed 10/11/15.

266.Wright WF, Oliverio JA. First Case of Lyme Arthritis Involving a Prosthetic Knee Joint. *Open Forum Infect Dis.* 2016;3(2):ofw096.

267. Cohen JR, Bradley AT, Lieberman JR. Preoperative Interventions and Charges Before Total Knee Arthroplasty. *J Arthroplasty*. 2016.

268. http://www.ixodes.ch. Last accessed 9/25/17.

269. Ixogel® is Granted QIDP Status by the US Food and Drug Administration press release released September 29,2015 at http://www.pr.com/press-release/639538. Last accessed 9/25/17.

270. Schwameis M, Kundig T, Huber G, et al. Topical azithromycin for the prevention of Lyme borreliosis: a randomised, placebo-controlled, phase 3 efficacy trial. *Lancet Infect Dis*. 2016.

271. Treatment & what has been overlooked so far at http://www.ixodes.ch/medical need.html. Last accessed 9/25/17.

272. Richard Louv, recipient of the Audobon Metal, author of the National BestSeller Last Child in the Woods at http://richardlouv.com/books/last-child/. Last accessed 9/24/17.

273. Bacon RM, Kugeler KJ, Mead PS. Surveillance for Lyme disease-- United States, 1992-2006. *MMWR Surveill Summ*. 2008;57(10):1-9.

274. Ogden NH, Bouchard C, Kurtenbach K, et al. Active and Passive Surveillance, and Phylogenetic Analysis of Borrelia burgdorferi Elucidate the Process of Lyme Disease Risk Emergence in Canada. *Environ Health Perspect*. 2010.

275. Xu G, Mather TN, Hollingsworth CS, Rich SM. Passive Surveillance of Ixodes scapularis (Say), Their Biting Activity, and Associated Pathogens in Massachusetts. *Vector Borne Zoonotic Dis*. 2016;16(8):520-527.

276. Daly ER, Fredette C, Mathewson AA, Dufault K, Swenson DJ, Chan BP. Tick bite and Lyme disease-related emergency department encounters in New Hampshire, 2010-2014. *Zoonoses Public Health*. 2017.

277. Sood SK. Lyme disease in children. *Infect Dis Clin North Am*. 2015;29(2):281-294.

278. Cook MJ. Lyme borreliosis: a review of data on transmission time after tick attachment. *Int J Gen Med.* 2015;8:1-8.

279. Blacklegged Ticks (Deer Tick, Bear Tick) from the University of Minnesota Department of Health at http://www.health.state.mn.us/divs/idepc/dtopics/tickborne/ticks.html. Last accessed 9/24/17.

280. Shadick NA, Zibit MJ, Nardone E, DeMaria A, Jr., Iannaccone CK, Cui J. A School-Based Intervention to Increase Lyme Disease Preventive Measures Among Elementary School-Aged Children. *Vector Borne Zoonotic Dis.* 2016;16(8):507-515.

281. Beaujean D, Crutzen R, Kengen C, van Steenbergen J, Ruwaard D. Increase in Ticks and Lyme Borreliosis, Yet Research into Its Prevention on the Wane. *Vector Borne Zoonotic Dis.* 2016;16(5):349-351.

282. Lantos PM, Lipsett SC, Nigrovic LE. False Positive Lyme Disease IgM Immunoblots in Children. *J Pediatr.* 2016.

283. Johnson L, Wilcox S, Mankoff J, Stricker RB. Severity of chronic Lyme disease compared to other chronic conditions: a quality of life survey. *PeerJ.* 2014;2.

284. Sharma A, Guleria S, Sharma R, Sharma A. Lyme Disease: A Case Report with Typical and Atypical Lesions. *Indian Dermatol Online J.* 2017;8(2):124-127.

285. Public Hearing of the State of Connecticut, Department of Public Health, In Re: Lyme Disease, held January 29, 2004 Hartford, Connecticut. at http://www.ct.gov/ag/lib/ag/health/0129lyme.pdf. Last accessed 12/31/15.

286. Nelson CA, Hayes CM, Markowitz MA, et al. The heat is on: Killing blacklegged ticks in residential washers and dryers to prevent tickborne diseases. *Ticks Tick Borne Dis.* 2016;7(5):958-963.

287. Carroll JF, Kramer M. Different activities and footwear influence exposure to host-seeking nymphs of Ixodes scapularis and

Amblyomma americanum (Acari: Ixodidae). *J Med Entomol.* 2001;38(4):596-600.

288. Jordan RA, Schulze TL, Dolan MC. Efficacy of plant-derived and synthetic compounds on clothing as repellents against Ixodes scapularis and Amblyomma americanum (Acari: Ixodidae). *J Med Entomol.* 2012;49(1):101-106.

289. Transmission from The Centers for Disease Control and Prevention, Reuters March 4, 2015, at https://www.cdc.gov/lyme/transmission/. Last accessed 3/24/17.

290. Shih CM, Telford SR, 3rd, Pollack RJ, Spielman A. Rapid dissemination by the agent of Lyme disease in hosts that permit fulminating infection. *Infect Immun.* 1993;61(6):2396-2399.

291. Goddard J. A ten-year study of tick biting in Mississippi: implications for human disease transmission. *J Agromedicine.* 2002;8(2):25-32.

292. Scoles GA, Papero M, Beati L, Fish D. A relapsing fever group spirochete transmitted by Ixodes scapularis ticks. *Vector Borne Zoonotic Dis.* 2001;1(1):21-34.

293. Krause PJ, Barbour AG. Borrelia miyamotoi: The Newest Infection Brought to Us by Deer Ticks. *Ann Intern Med.* 2015;163(2):141-142.

294. van Duijvendijk G, Coipan C, Wagemakers A, et al. Larvae of Ixodes ricinus transmit Borrelia afzelii and B. miyamotoi to vertebrate hosts. *Parasit Vectors.* 2016;9(1):97.

295. Tulane National Primate Research Center at http://www2.tulane.edu/tnprc/. Last accessed 3/22/17.

296. Ramesh G, Didier PJ, England JD, et al. Inflammation in the pathogenesis of lyme neuroborreliosis. *Am J Pathol.* 2015;185(5):1344-1360.

297. Kowarik MC, Cepok S, Sellner J, et al. CXCL13 is the major

determinant for B cell recruitment to the CSF during neuroinflammation. *J Neuroinflammation.* 2012;9:93.

298. Batheja S, Nields JA, Landa A, Fallon BA. Post-treatment lyme syndrome and central sensitization. *J Neuropsychiatry Clin Neurosci.* 2013;25(3):176-186.

299. Zimering JH, Williams MR, Eiras ME, Fallon BA, Logigian EL, Dworkin RH. Acute and chronic pain associated with Lyme borreliosis: clinical characteristics and pathophysiologic mechanisms. *Pain.* 2014;155(8):1435-1438.

300. Lopez-Sola M, Woo CW, Pujol J, et al. Towards a neurophysiological signature for fibromyalgia. *Pain.* 2016.

301. Glover GH. Overview of functional magnetic resonance imaging. *Neurosurg Clin N Am.* 2011;22(2):133-139, vii.

302. Researchers Discover 'Brain Signature' for Fibromyalgia by Pat Anson in Pain News Network on August 18, 2016

in http://www.painnewsnetwork.org/stories/2016/10/18/researchers-discover-brain-signature-for-fibromyalgia. Last accessed 10/22/16.

303. Breakthrough First Step in Brain-Based Fibromyalgia Diagnosis by Caitlyn Fitzpatrick in HCPlive on August 17, 2016

in http://www.hcplive.com/medical-news/breakthrough-first-step-in-brain-based-fibromyalgia-diagnosis. Last accessed 10/22/16.

304. Puri BK, Monro JA, Julu PO, Kingston MC, Shah M. Hyperosmia in Lyme disease. *Arq Neuropsiquiatr.* 2014;72(8):596-597.

305. Casselli T, Qureshi H, Peterson E, et al. MicroRNA and mRNA Transcriptome Profiling in Primary Human Astrocytes Infected with Borrelia burgdorferi. *PLoS One.* 2017;12(1):e0170961.

306. Gyllemark P, Forsberg P, Ernerudh J, Henningsson AJ. Intrathecal Th17- and B cell-associated cytokine and chemokine responses in

relation to clinical outcome in Lyme neuroborreliosis: a large retrospective study. *J Neuroinflammation.* 2017;14(1):27.

307. Harman MW, Hamby AE, Boltyanskiy R, et al. Vancomycin Reduces Cell Wall Stiffness and Slows Swim Speed of the Lyme Disease Bacterium. *Biophys J.* 2017;112(4):746-754.

308. Bruniera FR, Ferreira FM, Saviolli LR, et al. The use of vancomycin with its therapeutic and adverse effects: a review. *Eur Rev Med Pharmacol Sci.* 2015;19(4):694-700.

309. Schwan TG, Burgdorfer W, Schrumpf ME, Karstens RH. The urinary bladder, a consistent source of Borrelia burgdorferi in experimentally infected white-footed mice (Peromyscus leucopus). *J Clin Microbiol.* 1988;26(5):893-895.

310. Barthold SW, de Souza MS, Janotka JL, Smith AL, Persing DH. Chronic Lyme borreliosis in the laboratory mouse. *Am J Pathol.* 1993;143(3):959-971.

311. Moody KD, Barthold SW, Terwilliger GA, Beck DS, Hansen GM, Jacoby RO. Experimental chronic Lyme borreliosis in Lewis rats. *Am J Trop Med Hyg.* 1990;42(2):165-174.

312. Goodman JL, Jurkovich P, Kodner C, Johnson RC. Persistent cardiac and urinary tract infections with Borrelia burgdorferi in experimentally infected Syrian hamsters. *J Clin Microbiol.* 1991;29(5):894-896.

313. Preac Mursic V, Patsouris E, Wilske B, Reinhardt S, Gross B, Mehraein P. Persistence of Borrelia burgdorferi and histopathological alterations in experimentally infected animals. A comparison with histopathological findings in human Lyme disease. *Infection.* 1990;18(6):332-341.

314. Sonnesyn SW, Manivel JC, Johnson RC, Goodman JL. A guinea pig model for Lyme disease. *Infect Immun.* 1993;61(11):4777-4784.

315. Straubinger RK, Summers BA, Chang YF, Appel MJ. Persistence

of Borrelia burgdorferi in experimentally infected dogs after antibiotic treatment. *J Clin Microbiol.* 1997;35(1):111-116.

316. Roberts ED, Bohm RP, Jr., Cogswell FB, et al. Chronic lyme disease in the rhesus monkey. *Lab Invest.* 1995;72(2):146-160.

317. Hodzic E. Lyme Borreliosis: Is there a preexisting (natural) variation in antimicrobial susceptibility among Borrelia burgdorferi strains? *Bosn J Basic Med Sci.* 2015;15(3):1-13.

318. Hodzic E, Imai D, Feng S, Barthold SW. Resurgence of persisting non-cultivable Borrelia burgdorferi following antibiotic treatment in mice. *PLoS One.* 2014;9(1):e86907.

319. Biskup UG, Strle F, Ruzic-Sabljic E. Loss of plasmids of Borrelia burgdorferi sensu lato during prolonged in vitro cultivation. *Plasmid.* 2011;66(1):1-6.

320. Schwan TG, Burgdorfer W, Garon CF. Changes in infectivity and plasmid profile of the Lyme disease spirochete, Borrelia burgdorferi, as a result of in vitro cultivation. *Infect Immun.* 1988;56(8):1831-1836.

321. Stanek G, Strle F. Lyme borreliosis. *Lancet.* 2003;362(9396):1639-1647.

322. Hodzic E, Feng S, Holden K, Freet KJ, Barthold SW. Persistence of Borrelia burgdorferi following antibiotic treatment in mice. *Antimicrob Agents Chemother.* 2008;52(5):1728-1736.

323. Barthold SW, Hodzic E, Imai DM, Feng S, Yang X, Luft BJ. Ineffectiveness of tigecycline against persistent Borrelia burgdorferi. *Antimicrob Agents Chemother.* 2010;54(2):643-651.

324. Mali S, Mitchell M, Havis S, et al. A Proteomic Signature of Dormancy in an Actinobacterium: Micrococcus luteus. *J Bacteriol.* 2017.

325. Cunningham MEA, Doroshow R, Olivieri L, Moak JP. Junctional ectopic tachycardia secondary to myocarditis associated with sudden cardiac arrest. *HeartRhythm Case Rep.* 2017;3(2):124-128.

326.Bransfield RC. Suicide and Lyme and associated diseases. *Neuropsychiatr Dis Treat.* 2017;13:1575-1587.

327.Tager FA, Fallon BA, Keilp J, Rissenberg M, Jones CR, Liebowitz MR. A controlled study of cognitive deficits in children with chronic Lyme disease. *J Neuropsychiatry Clin Neurosci.* 2001;13(4):500-507.

328.Munir A, Aadil M, Rehan Khan A. Suicidal and homicidal tendencies after Lyme disease: an ignored problem. *Neuropsychiatr Dis Treat.* 2017;13:2069-2071.

329.Banerjee R, Liu JJ, Minhas HM. Lyme neuroborreliosis presenting with alexithymia and suicide attempts. *J Clin Psychiatry.* 2013;74(10):981.

330.Juchnowicz D, Rudnik I, Czernikiewicz A, Zajkowska J, Pancewicz SA. [Mental disorders in the course of lyme borreliosis and tick borne encephalitis]. *Przegl Epidemiol.* 2002;56 Suppl 1:37-50.

331.Bransfield RC. Author's reply. *Neuropsychiatr Dis Treat.* 2017;13:2071.

332.A single tick bite could put you at risk for at least 6 different diseases by Kevin Loria in Business Insider June 28, 2017 at http://www.businessinsider.com/deer-tick-can-carry-lyme-disease-powassan-virus-babesiosis-and-more-2017-6. Last accessed 7/2/17.

333.A little-known tick-borne infection could have permanent or fatal consequences by Kevin Loria in Business Insider June 27, 2017 at http://www.businessinsider.com/deer-tick-powassan-virus-lyme-disease-risk-2017-6. Last accessed 7/2/17.

334.Raileanu C, Moutailler S, Pavel I, et al. Borrelia Diversity and Co-infection with Other Tick Borne Pathogens in Ticks. *Frontiers in cellular and infection microbiology.* 2017;7:36.

335.Schouls LM, Van De Pol I, Rijpkema SG, Schot CS. Detection and identification of Ehrlichia, Borrelia burgdorferi sensu lato, and

Bartonella species in Dutch Ixodes ricinus ticks. *J Clin Microbiol.* 1999;37(7):2215-2222.

336. Nelder MP, Russell CB, Sheehan NJ, et al. Human pathogens associated with the blacklegged tick Ixodes scapularis: a systematic review. *Parasit Vectors.* 2016;9:265.

337. Knox KK, Thomm AM, Harrington YA, Ketter E, Patitucci JM, Carrigan DR. Powassan/Deer Tick Virus and Borrelia Burgdorferi Infection in Wisconsin Tick Populations. *Vector Borne Zoonotic Dis.* 2017.

338. Jones EH, Hinckley AF, Hook SA, et al. Pet ownership increases human risk of encountering ticks. *Zoonoses Public Health.* 2017.

339. Glanternik JR, Baine IL, Tormey CA, Rychalsky MR, Baltimore RS. A Cluster of Cases of Babesia Microti Among Neonates Traced to a Single Unit of Donor Blood. *Pediatr Infect Dis J.* 2017.

340. Saetre K, Godhwani N, Maria M, et al. Congenital Babesiosis After Maternal Infection With Borrelia burgdorferi and Babesia microti. *J Pediatric Infect Dis Soc.* 2017. .

341. Herrin BH, Peregrine AS, Goring J, Beall MJ, Little SE. Canine infection with Borrelia burgdorferi, Dirofilaria immitis, Anaplasma spp. and Ehrlichia spp. in Canada, 2013-2014. *Parasit Vectors.* 2017;10(1):244.

342. Kantamaneni V, Sunder V, Bilal M, Vargo S. A Case of Early Disseminated Neurological Lyme Disease Followed by Atypical Cutaneous Manifestations. *Case Rep Infect Dis.* 2017;2017:6598043.

343. Chaudhry MA, Satti SD, Friedlander IR. Lyme carditis with complete heart block: management with an external pacemaker. *Clin Case Rep.* 2017;5(6):915-918.

344. Parkitny L, Younger J. Reduced Pro-Inflammatory Cytokines after Eight Weeks of Low-Dose Naltrexone for Fibromyalgia. *Biomedicines.* 2017;5(2).

345. Cervantes J. Doctor says you are cured, but you still feel the pain. Borrelia DNA persistence in Lyme disease. *Microbes Infect.* 2017.

346. Livorsi D, Comer AR, Matthias MS, Perencevich EN, Bair MJ. Barriers to guideline-concordant antibiotic use among inpatient physicians: A case vignette qualitative study. *J Hosp Med.* 2016;11(3):174-180.

347. Koetsveld J, Draga ROP, Wagemakers A, et al. In vitro susceptibility of the relapsing fever spirochete Borrelia miyamotoi to antimicrobial agents. *Antimicrob Agents Chemother.* 2017.

348. Toussaint L, Sirois F, Hirsch J, et al. Gratitude mediates quality of life differences between fibromyalgia patients and healthy controls. *Qual Life Res.* 2017.

349. Stein E, Elbadawi LI, Kazmierczak J, Davis JP. Babesiosis Surveillance - Wisconsin, 2001-2015. *MMWR Morb Mortal Wkly Rep.* 2017;66(26):687-691.

350. Eickhoff C, Blaylock J. Tickborne diseases other than Lyme in the United States. *Cleve Clin J Med.* 2017;84(7):555-567.

351. Patel K, Shah S, Subedi D. Clinical association: Lyme disease and Guillain-Barre syndrome. *Am J Emerg Med.* 2017.

352. Bernard A, Kodjikian L, Abukhashabh A, et al. Diagnosis of Lyme-associated uveitis: value of serological testing in a tertiary centre. *Br J Ophthalmol.* 2017.

353. Powassan Virus from the Centers for Disease Control and Prevention at https://www.cdc.gov/powassan/index.html. Last accessed 9/14/17.

354. Powassan Virus from the Centers for Disease Control and Prevention from CNN at http://www.cnn.com/2017/05/03/health/powassan-tick-virus/index.html. Last accessed 9/14/17.

355. Frost HM, Schotthoefer AM, Thomm AM, et al. Serologic

Evidence of Powassan Virus Infection in Patients with Suspected Lyme Disease1. *Emerg Infect Dis.* 2017;23(8):1384-1388.

356. Permethrin Fact Sheet: Did you know? from the University of Rhode Island TickEncounter Resource Center at http://www.tickencounter.org/prevention/permethrin. Last accessed 9/14/17.

357. Eisen L, Rose D, Prose R, et al. Bioassays to evaluate non-contact spatial repellency, contact irritancy, and acute toxicity of permethrin-treated clothing against nymphal Ixodes scapularis ticks. *Ticks Tick Borne Dis.* 2017.

358. Health Effects of Permethrin-Impregnated Army Battle-Dress Uniforms (1994) by National Research Council. 1994. Washington, DC: The National Academies Press. https://doi.org/10.17226/9274. at https://www.nap.edu/catalog/9274/health-effects-of-permethrin-impregnated-army-battle-dress-uniforms. Last accessed 8/12/17.

359. Artal FJC. Infectious diseases causing autonomic dysfunction. *Clin Auton Res.* 2017.

360. Gila L, Guerrero A, Astarloa R, Marti P, Gutierrez JM. [Reflex sympathetic dystrophy. A new manifestation of Lyme disease?]. *Enferm Infecc Microbiol Clin.* 1990;8(1):32-35.

361. Bruckbauer HR, Preac Mursic V, Herzer P, Hofmann H. Sudeck's atrophy in Lyme borreliosis. *Infection.* 1997;25(6):372-376.

362. Neumann A, Schlesier M, Schneider H, Vogt A, Peter HH. Frequencies of Borrelia burgdorferi-reactive T lymphocytes in Lyme arthritis. *Rheumatol Int.* 1989;9(3-5):237-241.

363. Sibanc B, Lesnicar G. Complex regional pain syndrome and lyme borreliosis: two different diseases? *Infection.* 2002;30(6):396-399.

364. LeBel DP, 2nd, Moritz ED, O'Brien JJ, et al. Cases of transfusion-transmitted babesiosis occurring in nonendemic areas: a diagnostic dilemma. *Transfusion.* 2017.

365. Rashid AN, van Hensbroek MB, Kolader M, Hovius JW, Pajkrt D.

Lyme Borreliosis in Children: A Tertiary Referral Hospital Based Retrospective Analysis. *Pediatr Infect Dis J.* 2017.

366. Greenberg R. Chronic Lyme Disease: An Unresolved Controversy. *Am J Med.* 2017;130(9):e423.

367. Dall'Agnol B, Michel T, Weck B, et al. Borrelia burgdorferi sensu lato in Ixodes longiscutatus ticks from Brazilian Pampa. *Ticks Tick Borne Dis.* 2017.

368. Cameron D, Gaito A, Harris N, et al. Evidence-based guidelines for the management of Lyme disease. *Expert Rev Anti Infect Ther.* 2004;2(1 Suppl):S1-13.

369. Rhee H, Cameron DJ. Lyme disease and pediatric autoimmune neuropsychiatric disorders associated with streptococcal infections (PANDAS): an overview. *Int J Gen Med.* 2012;5:163-174.

370. Cameron DJ. Proof that chronic lyme disease exists. *Interdiscip Perspect Infect Dis.* 2010;Article ID 876450, 4 pages, doi:10.1155/2010/876450.

371. Cameron DJ. Insufficient evidence to deny antibiotic coverage to chronic Lyme disease patients. *Med Hypotheses.* 2009;72:688-691.

372. Cameron DJ. Clinical trials validate the severity of persistent Lyme disease symptoms. *Med Hypotheses.* 2008;72:153-156.

373. Cameron DJ. Generalizability in two clinical trials of Lyme disease. *Epidemiol Perspect Innov.* 2006;3:12.

PREVIEW NEXT BOOK.

There are more Inside Lyme books coming. Here are seven previews of upcoming chapters that are sure to be included in Dr. Cameron's next book.

PREVIEW 1: 12-YEAR-OLD BOY SUFFERS CARDIAC ARREST BECAUSE OF LYME DISEASE

In the February 2017 issue of *HeartRhythm Case Reports*, doctors describe what they believe is the first case of a Lyme disease patient presenting with fulminant myocarditis and cardiac arrest. Lyme disease has been associated with junctional ectopic tachycardia (JET) and fascicular tachycardia. In this instance, JET was secondary to fulminant myocarditis.

The patient is a 12-year-old previously healthy boy who had recently attended an outdoor camp for 2 to 3 weeks. He "began to gasp for air while riding as a passenger in a car, with subsequent cyanosis and cardiac arrest, following participation in recreational outdoor activities earlier that afternoon,"[325] state Cunningham and colleagues from the Division of Cardiology, Children's National Health System, Washington, D.C.

The boy received cardiopulmonary resuscitation for pulseless arrest and ventricular fibrillation. Spontaneous circulation returned "after 8 minutes of cardiopulmonary resuscitation, including defibrillation, intubation, and intravenous (IV) epinephrine and lidocaine administration," according to Cunningham and colleagues.[325]

He required intensive therapy in the pediatric intensive care unit for symptoms that included extreme hypoxemia, challenging ventilation, and persistent tachyarrhythmias including fascicular tachycardia. He was treated with high dose dopamine, norepinephrine, ceftriaxone, and procainamide. Procainamide was changed to amiodarone because of hypotension.

Serologic tests were remarkable for a strongly positive enzyme-linked immunosorbent assay (ELISA), as well as positive IgG antibodies and IgM western blot test for Lyme disease. Intravenous ceftriaxone was continued for 21 days, with normalization of his ejection fraction.

While the boy made a full recovery of cardiac functioning, he had neurologic injury that required long-term rehabilitation. Brain imaging revealed he suffered from a global cerebral edema and moderate hypoxic injury to the basal ganglia, hippocampi, and primary motor and visual cortices. The damage left the patient "with altered mental status, agitation, and dysautonomia," the authors explain.[325]

They did not address whether the neurologic symptoms could be caused by a persistent tickborne infection that had not resolved.

PREVIEW 2: BLOOD DONOR INFECTS PREMATURE INFANTS WITH BABESIA

*B*abesia is a parasite which infects red blood cells, causing symptoms similar to those seen with malaria. It's typically transmitted by a tick bite but can be acquired through contaminated blood transfusions. The disease can be extremely difficult to recognize in adults. Imagine the challenge of diagnosing it in premature infants.

A team of researchers at Yale School of Medicine describe three premature infants — all in one neonatal intensive care unit — who contracted Babesia from a single 24-year-old blood donor. The report was published in the *Pediatric Infectious Diseases Journal.*[339]

Babesia is a frightening infection, given that it can be unknowingly transmitted to multiple people through blood banks, which have no foolproof way of screening donors.

"Screening questionnaires are clearly insufficient given the growing number of cases of transfusion-transmitted babesiosis," writes Glanternik from the Division of Infectious Diseases, Department of Pediatrics at Yale School of Medicine.[339]

Transfusion-transmitted babesiosis

The 24-year-old donor from Connecticut was not recognized by the blood bank and "was deemed suitable for donation by the American Red Cross and his serology was negative for all FDA-mandated tests," Glanternik explains.

Three premature infants contracted Babesia from this donor, with two of the infants developing high-grade parasitemia (presence of parasites in the blood), according to Glanternik.[339] The parasitemia rose to a high of 13.4% and 12.5% for Infant A and B, respectively. Parasitemia peaked at 6.8% for Infant C.

All three premature infants were treated with a combination of azithromycin and atovaquone despite published recommendations for clindamycin and quinine.[70] "The stability of oral suspension [of quinine] using capsules is undetermined," explains Glanternik. "Furthermore, quinine's narrow therapeutic index and potential adverse effects limits its utility in treating small children."

The infants were treated for 14 days — longer than the 7-10 day recommendation described in the Infectious Diseases Society of America (IDSA) guidelines.[70]

However, more than a month (48 days) after treatment, one of the infants relapsed. There were no specific signs that could be attributed solely to babesiosis, explains Glanternik.[339] But a "routine blood smear demonstrated relapse with 1% parasitemia."

By day 9 of retreatment, the smear was negative. Treatment continued for a total of 23 days. None of the three premature infants required transfusions.

Authors warn of difficulties detecting Babesia in infants

"Clinicians should maintain a high index of suspicion for neonatal babesiosis in an infant who has received a transfusion because the clinical manifestations and concomitant lab abnormalities are non-specific and resemble those present in prematurity even in the absence of infection."[339]

Several additional questions are worth pursuing:

1. Would longer initial treatment have prevented a relapse for Infant C.
2. What are the consequences for infants if Babesia is not detected by thick smear?
3. How can doctors be sure their newborns are clear of Babesia after clearing parasitology with Babesia by blood smear?

PREVIEW 3: CONGENITAL TRANSMISSION OF BABESIOSIS: TWO CASE REPORTS

Congenital babesiosis is considered a rare disease with only nine cases reported in the U.S. - all in the northeastern region where babesiosis is endemic. Now, the authors of an article published in the *Journal of the Pediatric Infectious Diseases Society* [340] discuss two new cases of congenital babesiosis.

Congenital transmission has been described in 7 previous cases, in which the infants presented with fever, anemia, and thrombocytopenia, explains Saetre from Cohen Children's Medical Center in New Hyde Park, New York. [340]"They all required a blood transfusion."

But these are the first cases, to the authors' knowledge, in which the mother was diagnosed with Lyme disease prior to delivery and presumably had a subclinical infection with *Babesia microti*.

"We describe the cases of 2 infants with congenital babesiosis born to mothers with prepartum Lyme disease and subclinical *Babesia microti* infection," writes Saetre.[340]

Infant #1

The first infant, a 4 1/2-week-old male, presented with a fever of 101.7, sleepiness and periodic irritability. His mother had been diagnosed with Lyme disease during her third trimester at 32 weeks' gestation. She presented with an erythema migrans rash and was treated successfully with amoxicillin.

Testing of the infant included a blood smear which revealed 2% Parasitemia for *Babesia spp.* He was treated with atovaquone and azithromycin. The authors point out, "these agents were selected instead of clindamycin and quinine because of reports that they are tolerated better."[340]

The infant did not require a blood transfusion and was found to be seronegative for antibodies to *B. burgdorferi*, the causative agent for Lyme disease. At his 2-month follow-up visit, he was "clinically well, and his splenomegaly had resolved."

Infant #2

At 35 weeks' gestation, the mother developed fevers and myalgias. An erythema migrans rash appeared at 37 weeks' gestation, at which time she was treated with amoxicillin. The infant was born at 38 weeks and had no perinatal complications, according to the authors.

The 18-day-old female infant was initially asymptomatic despite a positive *B. microti* PCR assay, but "1 week later, she developed neutropenia and anemia," according to Saetre.[340]

She was hospitalized and treated with azithromycin and atovaquone. "Because of symptomatic anemia, including malaise, tachycardia, and pallor, a blood transfusion was given to her on day 2 [of her hospitalization]."

On day 4 due to a persistently elevated parasite level and falling hematocrit, she was prescribed clindamycin. And was treated with all 3 antimicrobials for 14 days. The infant also required a transfusion, while the first did not. Both developed low level Parasitemia, while 1 had symptomatic anemia.

Both infants were treated longer than the recommended 7 to 10 days by the *Infectious Diseases Society of America* (IDSA)[70] "because of concerns about possible impaired parasite clearance in neonates," writes Saetre.[340]

The clinical presentation of the 2 cases of congenital babesiosis described by Saetre was similar to the 7 cases described in the literature. "Each infant developed symptoms between 19 and 41 days of age and, at the time of presentation to medical attention, had fever, pallor, hemolytic anemia, and thrombocytopenia," explains Saetre[340] "Neutropenia was present also in the majority of cases, including both cases presented here."

The authors highlight the growing risk of Babesia, pointing out that "depending on the region in which it was contracted, 2% to 40% of patients with early Lyme disease are coinfected with babesiosis."

According to the authors, "A 2010 study that evaluated ticks from 2 locations within Westchester County, New York, where our hospital is located, found that at these locations, 3.6% and 22.4% of ticks were coinfected with *B. burgdorferi* and *B. microti*." [340]

The two congenital cases of Babesia described by Saetre and colleagues raises questions for doctors and their pregnant patients.

1. Could Babesia in the first and second trimester lead to complications or death in utero?
2. Would doctors recognize Babesia in a pregnant woman or infant without an erythema migrans rash?
3. Would the complications and need for a transfusion for the second infant have been prevented if the infant had been treated at the time of their first visit when the *B. microti* PCR assay was positive?
4. Should women presenting with Lyme disease during their pregnancy be treated with a regimen that is effective for both Lyme disease and Babesia?

PREVIEW 4: TRANSFUSION-TRANSMITTED BABESIOSIS POPPING UP IN MORE STATES

*B*abesia, a severe, potentially life-threatening illness, has been identified in as many as 40 percent of people with Lyme disease in the northeastern United States. The clinical spectrum now includes what has been described as "asymptomatic." This is particularly concerning given that the infection can be acquired not only through a tick bite but also through blood transfusions.

Transfusion-transmitted babesiosis (TTB) cases have been reported in Maryland, Nebraska, and South Carolina, and "serve as a reminder of the potential for TTB, especially in states not endemic for Babesia," cautions LeBel II and colleagues from the Department of Pathology and Laboratory Medicine at the Medical University of South Carolina.[364]

In their article published in the journal *Transfusion*, the authors report on two patients with TTB, identified as Cases 2 and 3. One patient was asymptomatic, and both lived in nonendemic states (Maryland and South Carolina).[364] The report highlights the difficulty of identifying the Babesia in blood supply by simply tracing the donors.

"The donor implicated in Cases 2 and 3 was a 30-year-old man residing in Maryland who denied any tick exposure; however, he had a history of Lyme disease and reported owning two dogs and traveling to coastal areas in Connecticut, Maryland, Massachusetts, New York, and Virginia in the past 2 years." This donor was positive by IFA and PCR 106 and 239 days after collection of implicated transfusions for Cases 2 and 3, respectively.[364]

These "asymptomatic" individuals challenge doctors in nonendemic areas of the United States. "Healthy, asymptomatic individuals and individuals without knowledge of babesiosis are at the highest risk for donating contaminated blood products," the authors point out.[364]

Universal screening of all blood donations in the United States has not been deemed cost effective, according to the authors. The risk of transfusion-transmitted babesiosis is expected to be reduced by screening blood in endemic states. However, this may not be effective because "blood products collected in Babesia-endemic areas are distributed nationally thus, clinicians in non-endemic states may fail to include babesiosis in the differential diagnosis of a patient who had a recent transfusion history and a fever of unknown origin," the authors explain.[364]

The article highlights the limitations of the questionnaire that blood banks provide to donors: The questionnaire assesses for babesiosis using the following question: "Have you ever had babesiosis?"[364]

PREVIEW 5: COULD AUTONOMIC DYSFUNCTION LEAD TO PAIN IN LYME DISEASE?

In his review of autonomic dysfunction caused by infectious diseases, Artal, from the Neurology Department at Raigmore Hospital in the United Kingdom, writes, "Complex regional pain syndromes [CRPS] and reflex sympathetic dystrophy with regional sympathetic hyperactivity have ... been reported in some patients with Lyme disease."[359]

The autonomic nervous system is responsible for control of bodily functions not consciously directed, such as breathing, the heartbeat, and digestive processes. Postural orthostatic tachycardia syndrome (POTS) is an example of autonomic dysfunction seen in Lyme disease. CRPS is characterized by considerable pain (allodynia, hyperalgesia), edema, and trophic changes of the skin and muscles.

Published in *Clinical Autonomic Research*, the article cites several cases,[360-363] including one in which a 46-year-old patient reported increasing pain and swelling in his left foot. The pain was so bad that his leg became dysfunctional, according to the authors. "Even the slightest contact with the skin of the affected area caused the patient unbearable pain."[359]

Another patient in one of the papers cited had been diagnosed with CRPS of unknown etiology for several months until he recalled having a tick bite on his left foot. He reported having a 5-cm erythema migrans (EM) rash, which disappeared over the next two weeks. He also had stiff muscles, a swollen knee, fatigue, depression, headaches, and bouts of dizziness. "On examination the patient presented with thickened upper part of his left foot which was diffusely painful to palpation. His left ankle was slightly swollen."[359]

"The borreliosis-associated etiology of CRPS in our patient was confirmed by the positive history of untreated erythema migrans (EM), oligoarthritis, positive serological tests for *B. burgdorferi* with seroconversion, detection of the *B. burgdorferi* genome in urine by PCR, as well as by the response to antibiotic therapy."[359]

The patient was prescribed a four-week course of ceftriaxone. After two weeks, he could stand on his foot without support. By the end of treatment, he could walk independently, the skin of the affected foot had resumed its normal appearance, and myalgia had vanished completely. The man was no longer depressed, and his headaches had disappeared. According to subjective evaluation, the pain was reduced by 75 percent, and therefore treatment was continued with doxycycline for another three weeks.[363]

Although less frequently than inflammatory and immune-mediated disorders, "infectious diseases may also affect the autonomic nervous system.

Artal points out that the pathogenesis of pain is unclear. However, "it is thought that complex regional pain could be either immune-mediated or due to the persistence of spirochete infection in the tissues."[359]

PREVIEW 6: CHRONIC LYME DISEASE: DOCTORS SEEK ANSWERS

In a 2017 issue of the *American Journal of Medicine*[366], Dr. Rosalie Greenberg from Overlook Hospital in Summit, N.J., responded to an article published by Drs. Shapiro, Baker and Wormser titled "False and Misleading Information about Lyme Disease."[203]

Greenberg's letter to the editor states, "The recently published article by Shapiro et al hoped to be topical in this age of 'alternative facts' but fell short, providing mainly biased viewpoints that prevent independent assessment of existing research in chronic Lyme disease. Presenting this conclusion as unquestionable is misleading."[366]

Shapiro and colleagues began their article as follows, "Recently, there has been considerable interest in the topic of fake news. For infectious diseases physicians, false and misleading information about the diagnosis and treatment of Lyme disease is not new. It is increasing in frequency and prominence, creating much confusion among primary care physicians and their patients."[203]

The authors dismiss the need for retreatment with antibiotics, stating, "results of multiple clinical trials show that patients with well-documented Lyme disease who have residual nonspecific symptoms after treatment do not benefit from additional treatment, even with extended courses of IV antibiotics."[203]

Greenberg's letter[366] expresses concern over the quality of data from the clinical trials cited by Shapiro and colleagues. Her concerns included the following: [203]

- "Critical statistical reviews of American antibiotic retreatment studies by more than one research group concluded that these trials were underpowered, did not prove that retreatment was ineffective, and found support for a possible role of antibiotics in retreatment of chronic Lyme disease."
- "Two trials demonstrated improvement in patients with severe significant symptoms at baseline."

In turn, Shapiro responded to Greenberg's letter, simply stating, "Most — if not all — of the issues raised by Greenberg in regards to our recent article have been addressed in detail in a previous publication in this journal."[203]

Greenberg concluded, "The authors' claim that definitive, rigorous, evidence based research exists regarding treatment of chronic Lyme disease is a disservice to fellow physicians and suffering patients alike. More and better-designed treatment studies in chronic Lyme disease are clearly needed."[366]

PREVIEW 7: CHILDREN IN THE NETHERLANDS ILL WITH POST-TREATMENT LYME BORRELIOSIS SYNDROME

Twelve out of 28 children with Lyme disease evaluated at an academic medical center in the Netherlands remained ill with post-treatment Lyme borreliosis syndrome (PTLBS). The 12 children presented with various complaints, including fatigue, general malaise, and pain. There were no other medical explanations for their complaints and all were positive for *Borrelia burgdorferi sensu lato* based on two-tier testing of C6 Lyme enzyme immunoassay (EIA) and IgG/IgM immunoblots.[365]

The authors conclude, however, that the symptoms were not caused by an active infection, since they lasted longer than six months. And therefore, the patients would not benefit from additional rounds of antibiotic treatment. "As more than 50% of the children had a duration of symptoms of more than 6 months, this further points towards other disorders than [Lyme borreliosis] eliciting the complaints of the studied patients," according to Rashid and colleagues from the Amsterdam Multidisciplinary Lyme Center located within the Academic Medical Center (AMC) in Amsterdam.[365]

The authors cite a 2015 article by Drs. Oliveira and Shapiro in support of their decision not to treat with antibiotics. "There is increasing evidence that viable *B. burgdorferi sensu lato* do not persist after conventional treatment with antimicrobials, which implies that persistent symptoms, after receiving conventional treatment for [Lyme borreliosis], should not be attributed to persistent active infection," the authors say. "Indeed, in our study only one patient was diagnosed with antibiotic refractory Lyme arthritis."[365]

Patients with early Lyme disease report having pain, fatigue, and post-treatment Lyme disease syndrome (PTLDS) following a three-week course of doxycycline, according to a study by Johns Hopkins University School of Medicine. Of 107 patients, 23 (21 percent) had a high fatigue score, 33 of the 107 patients (31 percent) had a high pain score, and six (6 percent) had PTLDS.[130]

In the John Hopkins' study, retreating patients with antibiotics was considered. "Of the 107 cases, 8 cases were re-treated with antibiotics after the initial three-week course of doxycycline because there was development of new objective findings (e.g., new neuropathy; 5 cases) or the EM rash did not fade after initial treatment or new rashes developed in other areas of the body (3 cases)," explain Bechtold and colleagues from the Department of Physical Medicine and Rehabilitation at Johns Hopkins University School of Medicine.[123]

It would be reasonable to look a second time at the children with PTLDS described in the Netherlands study to consider whether retreatment might be helpful.

ACKNOWLEDGMENTS

I am immensely grateful to Laurie Martin, my webmaster; Darlene Wood, my social media editor and expert; Sue Ferrara and Jean Pietrobono, my editors and contributors.

EDUCATIONAL VIDEOS BY DR. CAMERON

Dr. Cameron has produced four educational videos for his patients to begin their journey to understanding Lyme and tick-borne disease. The videos are under five minutes.

1. Lyme disease 101 - an introduction
2. Treatment decisions
3. Symptoms and manifestation of Lyme disease
4. Co-infections of Lyme disease

LYME DISEASE PATIENT PROFILES

Dr. Cameron has produced two educational videos for his patients understand Lyme disease from two patient's perspective. The videos are under five minutes.

1. Profiles in Lyme disease – Sophie
2. Profiles in Lyme disease - Ira

INSTAGRAM CONVERSATIONS

Dr. Daniel Cameron frequently posts on Lyme and related tick borne infections with his readers on instagram. Here are a few examples.

Can Lyme disease lead to a "new normal"?

Searching for the right diagnosis.

Personalized Lyme disease care planning

Ending "PTLDS": How Do We Get There From Here?

For more log onto instagram or my website.

through my website

through instagram

Feel free to log on to join the conversation.

FACEBOOK CONVERSATIONS

Dr. Daniel Cameron frequently posts on Lyme and related tick borne infections with his readers on Facebook. Here are a few examples.

Psychiatric symptoms are common in Lyme disease.

Fleeting lightheadedness and POTS associated with Lyme disease.

An astute mother led to the discovery of Lyme disease.

For more log onto facebook or my website.

through my website

through Facebook

Feel free to log on to join the conversation.

YOUTUBE CONVERSATIONS

Dr. Daniel Cameron frequently posts on Lyme and related tick borne infections with his readers on Youtube. Here are a few examples.

Boy suffers heart attack from Lyme Disease

Newborns contracted Babesia, a parasitic tick borne pathogen

Three Newborn children contract Babesia through blood transfusions

Good, bad, and ugly side of Post-Treatment-Lyme-Disease-Syndrome (PTLDS)

Dementia and Lyme disease

For more log onto facebook or my website.

through my website

through Youtube

. . .

Feel free to log on to join the conversation.

SELECTED RESEARCH BY DR. CAMERON

Evidence-based guidelines for the management of Lyme disease.[368]

Evidence assessments and guideline recommendations in Lyme disease: the clinical management of known tick bites, erythema migrans rashes and persistent disease.[69]

Lyme disease and pediatric autoimmune neuropsychiatric disorders associated with streptococcal infections (PANDAS): an overview.[369]

Proof that chronic Lyme disease exists.[370]

Insufficient evidence to deny antibiotic treatment to chronic Lyme disease patients[371]

Clinical trials validate the severity of persistent Lyme disease symptoms.[372]

Severity of Lyme disease with persistent symptoms. Insights from a double-blind placebo-controlled clinical trial[126]

Consequences of treatment delay in Lyme disease[148]

Generalizability in two clinical trials of Lyme disease[373]

LINKS TO READING RESOURCES

When writing a book to reach a variety of audience members—from patients to physicians to researchers to caregivers—one realizes some readers would benefit from additional information in order to understand passages.

There was thought here of creating a Glossary of Terms and an Appendix listing the various ticks and the infections they can potentially transmit. But then, the book would become even longer; and the writer puzzled what terms would need defining? Should there be pictures of ticks?

Consequently, the decision was made to provide readers the URL'S for websites which they could access when needed.

Medical Definitions:

Merriam-Webster Medical Dictionary: https://www.merriam-webster.com/medical

US National Library of Medicine-Medical Encyclopedia https://medlineplus.gov/encyclopedia.html

Tick Identification:

The University of Rhode Island TickEncounter Resource Center
http://www.tickencounter.org/

Tick ID section: http://www.tickencounter.org/tick_identification

Diseases:

CDC Tickborne Diseases of the United States

https://www.cdc.gov/ticks/diseases/index.html

Made in the USA
Las Vegas, NV
14 August 2023